Management of Common Gynecological Problems
A Guide for Practitioners

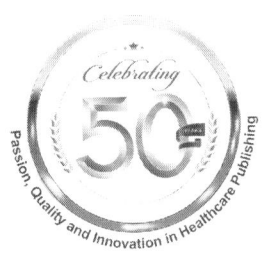

Management of Common Gynecological Problems
A Guide for Practitioners

Consulting Editor
Kanwal Gujral
DGO MS (Obs & Gyne) FICOG FIMSA FICMCH
Co-Chairperson and Senior Consultant
Institute of Obstetrics and Gynecology
Sir Ganga Ram Hospital
New Delhi, India

Series Editors

Atul Kakar
FRCP
Senior Consultant Physician and Rheumatologist
Vice Chairman
Department of Internal Medicine
Sir Ganga Ram Hospital
New Delhi, India

Samiran Nundy
MA MChir FRCP FRCS
Emeritus Consultant
Department of Surgical Gastroenterology and Liver Transplantation
Sir Ganga Ram Hospital
New Delhi, India

Foreword
Atul Kakar
Samiran Nundy

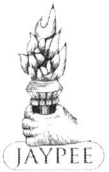

JAYPEE BROTHERS MEDICAL PUBLISHERS
The Health Sciences Publisher
New Delhi | London | Panama

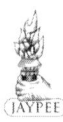 **Jaypee Brothers Medical Publishers (P) Ltd**

Headquarters
Jaypee Brothers Medical Publishers (P) Ltd
4838/24, Ansari Road, Daryaganj
New Delhi 110 002, India
Phone: +91-11-43574357
Fax: +91-11-43574314
E-mail: jaypee@jaypeebrothers.com

Overseas Offices

JP Medical Ltd
83 Victoria Street, London
SW1H 0HW (UK)
Phone: +44 20 3170 8910
Fax: +44 (0)20 3008 6180
E-mail: info@jpmedpub.com

Jaypee-Highlights Medical Publishers Inc
City of Knowledge, Bld. 235, 2nd Floor, Clayton
Panama City, Panama
Phone: +1 507-301-0496
Fax: +1 507-301-0499
E-mail: cservice@jphmedical.com

Jaypee Brothers Medical Publishers (P) Ltd
Bhotahity, Kathmandu, Nepal
Phone: +977-9741283608
E-mail: kathmandu@jaypeebrothers.com

Website: www.jaypeebrothers.com
Website: www.jaypeedigital.com

© 2019, Jaypee Brothers Medical Publishers

The views and opinions expressed in this book are solely those of the original contributor(s)/author(s) and do not necessarily represent those of editor(s) of the book.

All rights reserved. No part of this publication may be reproduced, stored or transmitted in any form or by any means, electronic, mechanical, photocopying, recording or otherwise, without the prior permission in writing of the publishers.

All brand names and product names used in this book are trade names, service marks, trademarks or registered trademarks of their respective owners. The publisher is not associated with any product or vendor mentioned in this book.

Medical knowledge and practice change constantly. This book is designed to provide accurate, authoritative information about the subject matter in question. However, readers are advised to check the most current information available on procedures included and check information from the manufacturer of each product to be administered, to verify the recommended dose, formula, method and duration of administration, adverse effects and contraindications. It is the responsibility of the practitioner to take all appropriate safety precautions. Neither the publisher nor the author(s)/editor(s) assume any liability for any injury and/or damage to persons or property arising from or related to use of material in this book.

This book is sold on the understanding that the publisher is not engaged in providing professional medical services. If such advice or services are required, the services of a competent medical professional should be sought.

Every effort has been made where necessary to contact holders of copyright to obtain permission to reproduce copyright material. If any have been inadvertently overlooked, the publisher will be pleased to make the necessary arrangements at the first opportunity. The **CD/DVD-ROM** (if any) provided in the sealed envelope with this book is complimentary and free of cost. **Not meant for sale.**

Inquiries for bulk sales may be solicited at: jaypee@jaypeebrothers.com

Management of Common Gynecological Problems: A Guide for Practitioners

First Edition: **2019**
ISBN: 978-93-5270-687-7
Printed at Replika Press Pvt. Ltd.

Contributors

Abha Majumdar

Anurag Vashista

Chandra Mansukhani

Debasis Dutta

Divya

Geeta Mediratta

Harsha Khullar

Indrani Ganguli

Kanika Chopra

Kanika Jain

Kanwal Gujral

Mala Srivastava

Mamta Dagar

Neeti Tiwari

Pallavi Sharma

Pramod Yerne

Punita Bhardwaj

Rakesh Kumar Koul

Rashmi Nigam

Ruma Satwik

Sharmistha Garg

Shweta Mittal Gupta

Foreword

Medicine is an ever-changing field. It is constantly advancing and the guidelines for practice keep altering so that busy practitioners find themselves lost and confused. This practitioners' series at the Ganga Ram Institute for Postgraduate Medical Education and Research is an attempt to inform the General and Family Physician what he or she needs to know. These books provide guidance on how to manage commonly encountered clinic situations in a simple and easy-to-understand language. We are sure that after going through this book readers will become more confident to tackle problems they meet every day.

Puberty and adolescence are important topic rarely discussed. The changes during this period are so intense that they require especially mention. The transition into adulthood has physiological, emotional and hormonal effects and they may impact social adjustment and a person's self-esteem.

Vaginal discharge is a common complaint in gynecological outpatient departments. Physicians need to differentiate between a normal and abnormal discharge and treat both appropriately. The other interesting, yet less discussed, topics are urinary problems in women. One chapter lists the common conditions responsible and their management. Pain in the pelvic region can very annoying and many chapters are dedicated to symptoms, i.e. chronic pelvic pain, pelvic inflammatory pain and dysmenorrhea.

These books we hope will serve as ready reckoners for practicing gynecologists and deal with all the changes between puberty and menopause. Their contents are written in simple english, so that comprehension is easy with many figures and illustrations to supplement the text. Breast, ovarian, cervical and endometrial cancers have been discussed with up-to-date information as is the vaccine for human papilloma and other preventive measures in gynecological practice.

We hope that our readers will find the publication a useful guide in their day-to-day work and would be pleased to receive feedback on how it might be improved.

Series Editors
Atul Kakar
Samiran Nundy

Preface

This book brings together contributions from experts on commonly encountered gynecological conditions, presenting pathophysiology, symptomatology and management in an easy-to-comprehend manner. All chapters liberally employ tables, original pictures/diagrams to enlist and explain important concepts.

The inaugural chapter deals with the physiology behind puberty and lists points to identify, investigate and manage girls presenting with abnormal puberty. The subsequent chapters deal with common conditions of menopause and vaginal discharge and help differentiate between normal symptoms from the abnormal. Dysmenorrhea and chronic pelvic pain can often be debilitating symptoms leading to loss of productive hours. Its management is detailed in the next two chapters. Urologists have often managed urinary problems in women. This book has a chapter presenting information on what a gynecologist ought to know and what do when she sees a patient with such a complaint.

All fibroids or ovarian cysts do not need medical or surgical intervention. Chapters 8 and 9 provide a closer insight into what needs attention and what can be left. Pelvic inflammatory disease has implications on a woman's well-being and reproduction. Chapter 10 details the symptomatology, investigations and management of pelvic inflammatory disease (PID).

The following chapter, explains how polycystic ovary syndrome (PCOS), the commonest endocrinological disorder in women, can manifest across all age groups in different ways and how best to manage it. The prevalence of infertility seems to be growing in women across the globe, largely due to delayed child-bearing but also due to fast-changing lifestyles, environmental pollutants and increasing work-related stress. Its work-up and management is dealt with in the next chapter.

The other end of the spectrum is contraception. In a country such as India, slated to be the world's most populous by 2030, safe, effective, cheap and readily acceptable contraceptive methods are the need of the hour. The chapter on contraception talks about what is on offer and for whom. Increasingly, the medical fraternity is moving from surgical abortion to the medical means. The do's and don'ts of medical abortion are dealt with next.

Two chapters in the book deal with abnormal postmenopausal bleeding and the burning question of whether hormone replacement therapy is safe and effective in postmenopausal women.

Prevention strategies employing early detection of that dreadful disease, cancer, can limit the morbidity and mortality associated with it. This is addressed in Chapters 15 and 16 followed by chapters on comprehensive surgical and medical-oncological management once the diagnosis is made.

It is hoped, that through this effort, general practitioners will find a readily usable and easy to understand reference book for common gynecological problems.

Kanwal Gujral

Acknowledgment

No book gets completed without help from its authors and I would especially like to thank ours for the efforts they made and the quality of their contributions to this volume. I am also grateful for the encouragement and support given to us by Professor Dr DS Rana, Chairman, Board of Management and Professor Dr Kusum Verma, Dean, GRIPMER (The Ganga Ram Institute for Postgraduate Medical Education and Research) who are always there behind us during all educational activities. I also thank Professors Atul Kakar and Samiran Nundy whose idea it was to start the GRIPMER Medical Series and push us towards completing this book in time.

Dr Lipika Khurana, Research Officer, from the obstetrics and gynecology office and Mr Parmanand Tiwari, Junior Executive in our hospital have helped us right from the beginning up to the completion of this important publication.

I greatly appreciate the staff of M/s Jaypee Brothers Medical Publishers (P) Ltd, New Delhi, India, for their assistance, thoroughness, patience and professional work.

I am thankful to Shri Jitendar P Vij (Group Chairman), Mr Ankit Vij (Managing Director), Ms Chetna Malhotra Vohra (Associate Director—Content Strategy), and Ms Payal Bharti (Senior Manager—Professional Publishing) of M/s Jaypee Brothers Medical Publishers (P) Ltd, New Delhi, India, for giving a go-ahead at the very beginning and helping us in every way possible to bring out this book.

Kanwal Gujral

Contents

1. **Normal and Abnormal Puberty** 1
   Chandra Mansukhani, Rashmi Nigam, Divya, Pallavi Sharma

   Puberty *1*
   - Mechanism *1*
   - Factors Determining Onset of Puberty *1*
   - Endocrinology in Puberty *2*
   - Thelarche and Adrenarche *4*
   - Changes in Genital Organs *4*
   - Delayed Puberty or Interrupted Puberty *6*
   - Precocious Puberty *9*

2. **Menopause: Physiology and Symptomatology** 15
   Mala Srivastava, Mamta Dagar
   - Premature Ovarian Failure *15*
   - Physiology *15*
   - Lipids and Lipoproteins *17*
   - Central Nervous System *17*
   - Prediction of Menopause *18*
   - Evaluation of the Women *18*
   - Sequelae of Ovarian Failure *20*

3. **Vaginal Discharge: Normal and Abnormal** 24
   Mala Srivastava
   - Normal Vaginal Discharge *24*
   - Natural Defense Mechanism of Vagina *25*
   - Flora Normally Present in Vagina *25*
   - Organisms Normally Present in the Vagina *25*
   - Causes of Vaginal Discharge *26*
   - Abnormal Vaginal Discharge *26*
   - Bacterial Vaginosis *28*
   - Fungal Infection *30*
   - Trichomoniasis *31*
   - *Neisseria Gonorrhoeae* *32*
   - Chlamydiasis *33*
   - Summary of Characteristics of Common Vaginal Infections *33*

4. **Abnormal Uterine Bleeding** 35
   Chandra Mansukhani, Anurag Vashista, Rashmi Nigam
   - Incidence *35*

- Etiology 35
- Approach to Abnormal Uterine Bleeding 36

5. **Dysmenorrhea** 49
   Punita Bhardwaj
   - Prevalence 49
   - Types 49
   - Etiology 50
   - Symptoms 54
   - Diagnosis 55
   - Treatment 56

6. **Chronic Pelvic Pain** 58
   Shweta Mittal Gupta
   - History 58
   - Causes of Chronic Pelvic Pain 59
   - Physical Examination 60
   - Diagnostic Test 62
   - Management 63

7. **Urinary Problems in Women: Hush No More** 67
   Geeta Mediratta
   - Urinary Incontinence 67
   - Types of Disorders 67
   - Risk Factors for Urinary Incontinence 69
   - Approach to Patient with Incontinence 69
   - Nonsurgical Treatment 72
   - Surgical Treatment for Stress Incontinence 74
   - Surgical Treatment for Detrusor Overactivity 75
   - Surgical Treatment of Fistula 75
   - Voiding Dysfunction 76
   - Bladder Pain Syndromes 77

8. **Fibroids: A Close Insight** 80
   Kanwal Gujral, Pramod Yerne, Anurag Vashista
   - Risk Factors 80
   - Signs and Symptoms 80
   - Classification 81
   - Diagnosis 81
   - Management of Fibroids 82

9. **When to Intervene in a Case of Ovarian Cyst?** 90
   Kanika Jain, Kanika Chopra
   - Functional Ovarian Cysts 90
   - Benign Ovarian Neoplasm 91

- Malignant Ovarian Neoplasm *93*
- Approach to the Patient with Ovarian Cyst *94*

10. Pelvic Inflammatory Disease 99
Kanwal Gujral
- Risk Factors for Pelvic Inflammatory Disease *99*
- Acute Pelvic Inflammatory Disease *99*

11. The Enigma of Polycystic Ovarian Syndrome 107
Ruma Satwik
- Definition and Diagnosis *107*
- Criteria in Adolescence *108*
- Management *114*

12. Management of an Infertile Couple 124
Abha Majumdar, Neeti Tiwari
- Evaluation of Female Partner *124*
- Evaluation of Male Partner *130*
- Treatment of Specific Disorders *133*
- Unexplained Infertility *139*

13. Contraception: Making the Right Choices 141
Mamta Dagar
- Contraceptive Choices and Efficacy *141*

14. Medical Abortion: What a General Practitioner Should Know? 156
Sharmistha Garg
- Clinical Care of the Women Undergoing Abortions *161*
- Medical Methods of Abortion—Adapted from World Health Organization Safe Abortion Guidelines 2012 *162*
- Complications of Abortions *163*

15. Breast Cancer Surveillance 165
Debasis Dutta, Kanika Chopra
- Breast Anatomy *165*
- Patients History and Physical Examination *165*
- Types of Lesions in Breast *167*
- Breast Cancer *167*

16. Screening of Gynecological Cancers 174
Indrani Ganguli
- Cervical Cancer *175*
- Breast Cancer *177*
- Ovarian Cancer *180*
- Endometrial Cancer *183*

- Vulvar Cancer *184*
- Vaginal Cancer *184*

17. Bleeding after Menopause 186
Harsha Khullar
- Causes of Bleeding *186*
- Management of Patients with Postmenopausal Bleeding *189*

18. Hormone Replacement Therapy in Menopause 193
Indrani Ganguli
- Myth of Menopause *193*
- Ancient India *194*
- Crisis of Menopausal Hormone Therapy *194*
- MHT and Urogynecology *197*
- Breast Cancer and MHT *197*
- MHT and Ovarian Cancer *198*
- Rationality of Low-dose MHT *198*
- Estrogen Replacement Therapy Newer Developments *200*
- Individualizing MHT *202*

19. Ovarian Cancer 204
Harsha Khullar
- Incidence *204*
- Classification *204*
- High Risk Factors *205*
- Epithelial Ovarian Tumor *205*
- Current Recommendations for Women at High Risk of Ovarian Cancer *206*
- Management *207*
- Follow-up after Treatment *207*
- Nonepithelial Ovarian Cancer *207*
- Management of Malignant Germ Cell Neoplasm *208*

20. Cervical Cancer 209
Mala Srivastava
- Epidemiology of Cancer Cervix *209*
- Mechanism of Carcinogens *209*
- Local Examination *210*
- Features of Carcinoma Cervix on Colposcopy *210*
- International Federation of Gynecology and Obstetrics (FIGO) Staging of Cancer of the Cervix Uteri (November 2018) *210*
- FIGO Staging of Carcinoma of the Cervix Uteri (2008) *211*
- Types of Cancer Cervix *212*
- Management of Invasive Cancer of the Cervix *213*

21. Cancer of Endometrium 221
Mamta Dagar
- Epidemiology *221*
- Histopathology *221*
- Risk Factors *222*
- Staging and Treatment *222*
- Pattern of Recurrence *225*
- Follow-up Care *227*
- Prognosis *227*

22. Management of Breast Cancer: An Overview 230
Rakesh Kumar Koul
- Symptoms *230*
- Evaluation of Breast Malignancy *230*
- Histology *231*
- Further Clinical Staging *232*
- Breast Cancer Staging *233*
- Molecular Profiling Assays *237*
- Management of Preinvasive Breast Tumors (Stage 0) *238*
- Treatment of Early Stage Invasive Breast Cancer *239*
- Locally Advanced Breast Cancers *244*
- Inflammatory Breast Cancer *244*
- Principles of Preoperative Systemic Therapy *244*
- Breast Reconstruction Following Surgery *245*
- Metastatic/Recurrent Breast Cancer *246*
- Fertility and Birth Control *248*

Index *251*

Plate 4

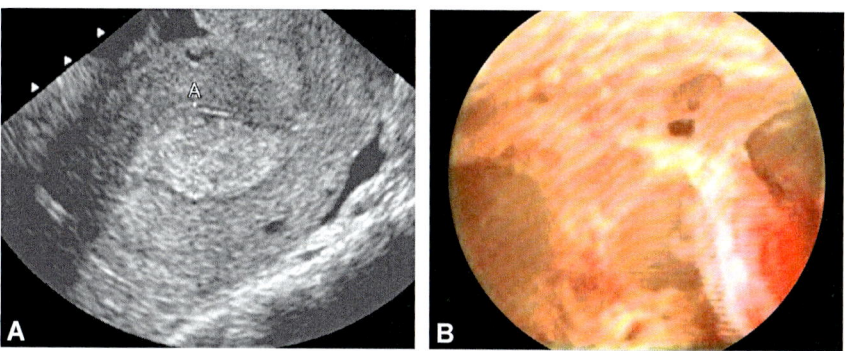

Figs. 17.3A and B: (A) Ultrasonography of hyperplasia; (B) Hysteroscopy of hyperplasia.

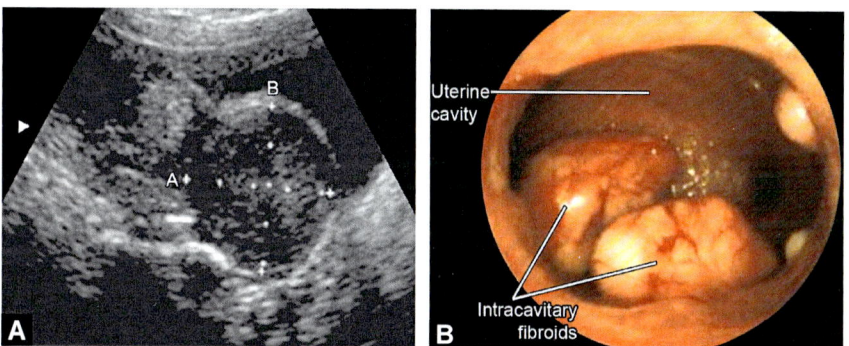

Figs. 17.4A and B: (A) Ultrasonography of fibroid; (B) Hysteroscopy of fibroid.

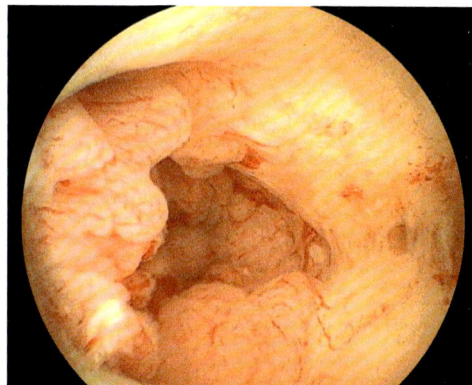

Fig. 17.5: Hysteroscopy of endometrial cancer.

Plate 3

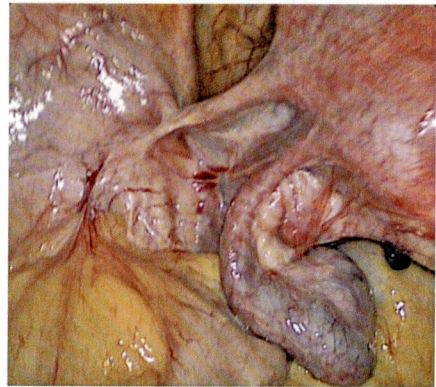

Fig. 10.2: Laparoscopy picture tubo-ovarian adhesions.

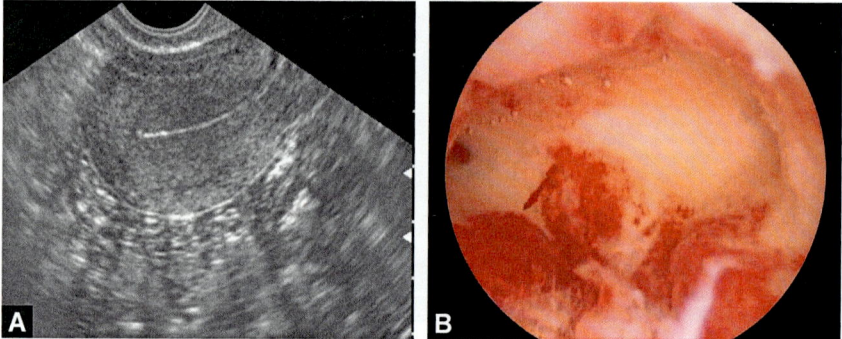

Figs. 17.1A and B: (A) Ultrasonography of vaginal atrophy;
(B) Hysteroscopy of vaginal atrophy.

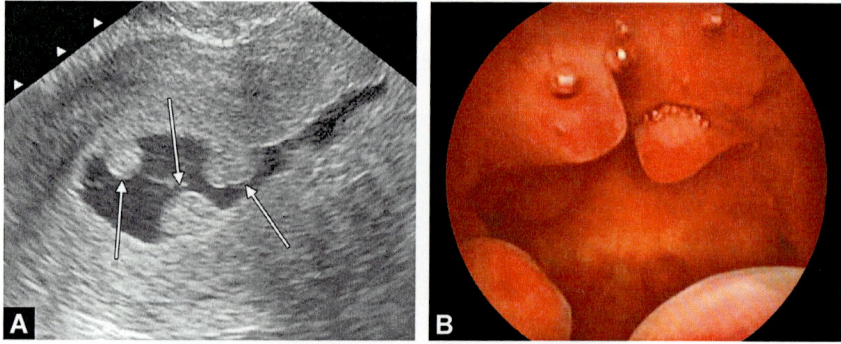

Figs. 17.2A and B: (A) Ultrasonography of uterine polyps;
(B) Hysteroscopy of uterine polyps.

Plate 2

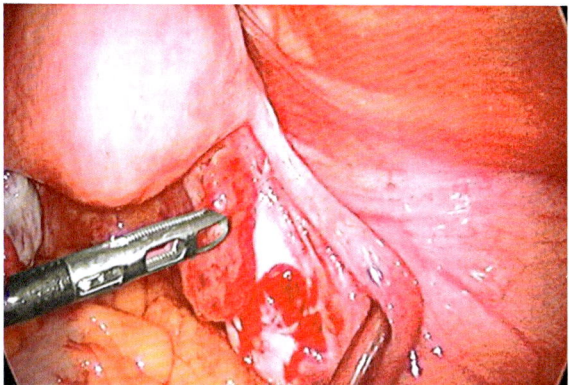

Fig. 9.1: Functional cyst seen in ovary.

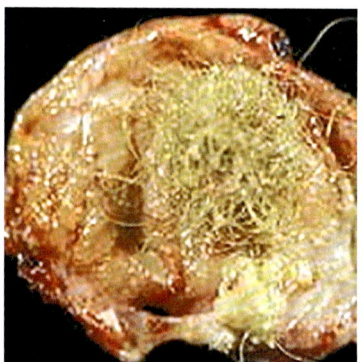

Fig. 9.2: Cut section image of a dermoid cyst.

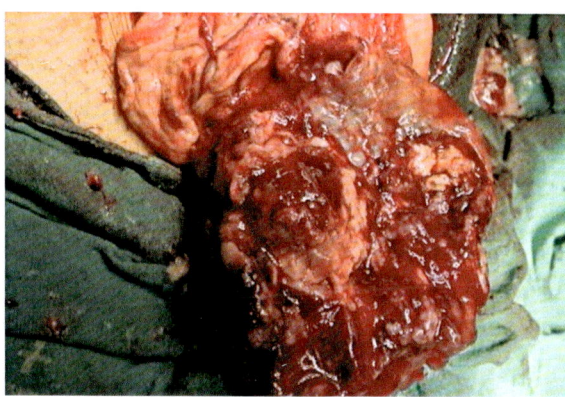

Fig. 9.3: Rare presentation of ruptured malignant germ cell tumor in a 12-year-old girl.

Plate 1

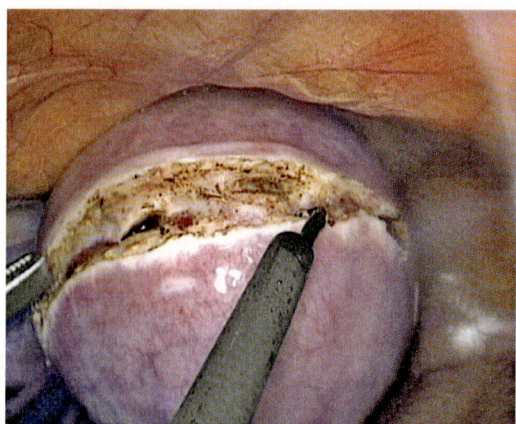

Fig. 8.3A: Laparoscopic myomectomy shows incision on myoma.

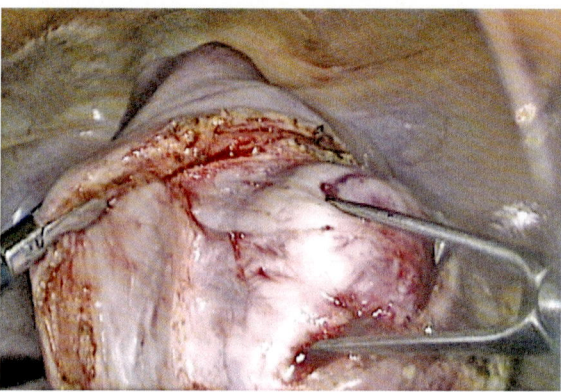

Fig. 8.3B: Laparoscopic myomectomy shows enucleation of myoma.

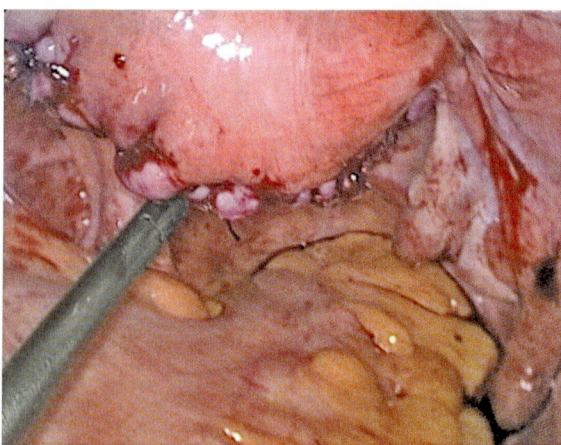

Fig. 8.3C: Laparoscopic myomectomy shows closure of myoma bed.

CHAPTER 1

Normal and Abnormal Puberty

Chandra Mansukhani, Rashmi Nigam, Divya, Pallavi Sharma

PUBERTY

DEFINITION

Puberty is defined as predictable sequence of events that occur over a fixed time period in which there is development of secondary sexual characteristics and reproductive function.

MECHANISM

The changes begin from 10 years of age and are completed by 16 years of age. Central nervous system (CNS) plays a pivotal role in initiating a cascade of events necessary for pubertal development. The interplay of hormones involved in the hypothalamus-pituitary-ovarian (H-P-O) axis an important event.

Before the onset of puberty the gonadotropins and gonadal steroids are in very low levels. This occurs as a result of negative feedback effect of estrogen to the hypothalamic pituitary system. But as puberty approaches, first there is increased pulsatile pattern of luteinizing hormone (LH) release in sleep followed by similar increased pulsatile but low amplitude LH release throughout 24 hours resulting in episodic peak levels of estradiol which bring about menstruation. Finally, there is establishment of positive feedback relationship between estradiol and LH leading to ovulatory cycles.

FACTORS DETERMINING ONSET OF PUBERTY

- *Genetics:* There exists a correlation between the age of menarche of mother, her female children and in sisters also.
- *Nutrition:* Improved nutrition and healthy life style has resulted in early age of menarche. Moderate obesity in young girls (20–30% of normal weight) results in early menarche, while morbid obesity (> 30% of normal

weight) would lead to delayed menarche. Severely malnourished girls, diabetics, normal weight girls who exercise intensely experience delayed menarche too.
- *Geography:* Children being closer to equator, low altitude areas, urban areas experience early menarche, than those being away from equator in high altitude and rural region.
- *Exposure to height:* Plays some role in time of menarche.
- Exposure to exogenous estrogens leads to early menarche.

ENDOCRINOLOGY IN PUBERTY

- *Hypothalamic-pituitary-ovarian axis (Flowchart 1.1):* The tonic and episode secretion of gonadotropins in prepubertal period is gradually changed to one of cyclic release in post pubertal period.
- Thyroid gland —has an important role in the H-P-O axis.
- *Hypothalamic-pituitary-ovarian axis:* [Gonadotropin-releasing hormone (GnRH)—follicle-stimulating hormone (FSH), LH —estradiol]. Levels of the gonadotropins and sex hormones remain at low level during initial few week of life and prepubertal period. However at the onset of puberty, even before the appearance of physical changes, there is increased sensitivity of LH to GnRH and increase in both FSH and LH levels during sleep. This is followed by increased secretion of estradiol, thus as puberty progresses, there is increase in basal levels of both FSH and LH and release becomes pulsatile.
- *Adrenal androgens:* There is increased production of androstenedione, dehydroepiandrosterone and its sulfate (DHEAS), the accelerated increase occurs 2 years before the increase in gonadotropins and gonadal sex steroid hormones. They are responsible for increased sebum production, development of hair in axillae and pubic area and voice changes.
- *Gonadal sex steroids:* Estradiol, predominantly produced by ovaries steadily increases during puberty, while estrone which is secreted partly by ovaries and partly due to conversion of estradiol and androstenedione

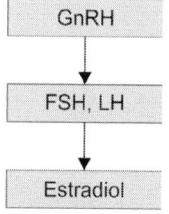

Flowchart 1.1: Hypothalamic-pituitary-ovarian axis.

(GnRH: gonadotropin-releasing hormone; FSH: follicle-stimulating hormone; LH: luteinizing hormone).

increases early in puberty but plateaus by mid puberty. Thus there is decrease in estrone to estradiol ratio as the puberty progresses. Gonadal estrogen leads to development of uterus, vagina and the breasts. They also have a direct effect on bone growth and height gain achieved by epiphyseal fusion.

- *Growth hormone:* At the onset of puberty, there is also a pulsatile secretion of growth hormone of high amplitude especially during sleep. The increase is mediated by estrogen. In girls the basal level of growth hormone (GH) remains high throughout puberty, reaching peak at the time of menarche and declining thereafter. GH exerts its action through insulin-like growth factor I (IGF-I). IGF-I is produced in almost all tissues with main source as liver.
- *Leptin:* A peptide secreted in adipose tissue acts on CNS determines eating behavior and energy balance. It is observed levels in patients with early menarche.
- *Thyroid gland:* Plays an important role in the H-P-O axis.

The sequences in which the changes of puberty occur (Flowchart 1.2).

- *Growth:* In girls the spurt occurs 2 years earlier (11–12 years) than in boys.
    - On an average, the growth peak is reached about 2 years after breast changes and approximately 1 year before menarche.
    - Estrogen along with GH and IGF-1 play together to bring about growth acceleration. It is important to note that adrenal androgens are not involved in growth.

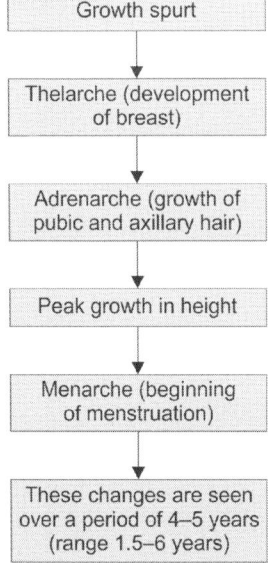

Flowchart 1.2: The sequences in which the changes of puberty occur.

- Skeletal age is more closely related to pubertal stage than with chronologic age.
- Estrogens are also involved in increase in total body fat and its peculiar distribution over the thighs, buttocks and abdomen.

THELARCHE AND ADRENARCHE

It can be described by Tanner staging (Tables 1.1 and 1.2) (Figs. 1.1 and 1.2).

CHANGES IN GENITAL ORGANS

Ovaries

- It becomes bulky and oval due to follicular enlargement and stromal cells proliferation.
- Uterine body and the cervix ration become 1:1 at menarche from 1:2 at birth and thereafter is enlargement of uterine body with ratio of 2:1.

Table 1.1: Thelarche and adrenarche are described by Tanner staging.

	Breast	Pubic hair
Stage I	Elevation of papilla only	No pubic hair present
Stage II	Breasts buds appears, papilla slightly elevated areola begins to enlarge (median age—9.8 years)	Sparse long hair on either side of labia majora (median age—10.5 years)
Stage III	Further growth of entire breast	Darker, coarse and curly hair over mons pubis
Stage IV	Secondary mound of areola and papilla projecting above the breast tissue (median age—12.1 years)	Adult type hair covering the mons only (median age—12 years)
Stage V	Areola recessed to general contour of breast (median age—14.6 years)	Adult hair with inverse triangle distribution covering the medial thigh (median age—13.7 years)

Table 1.2: Blood hormone concentrations during female puberty.

Tanner stage	FSH IU/L	LH IU/L	Estradiol pg/mL	DHA ng/dL
1	0.9–5.1	1.8–9.2	<10	19–302
2	1.4–7.0	2–16.6	7–37	45–1904
3	2.4–7.7	5.6–13.6	9–59	125–1730
4	1.5–11.2	7–14.4	10–156	153–134
Adult follicular	3–20	5–25	30–100	162–1620

(FSH: follicle-stimulating hormone; LH: luteinizing hormone; DHA: dehydroepiandrosterone).

Normal and Abnormal Puberty

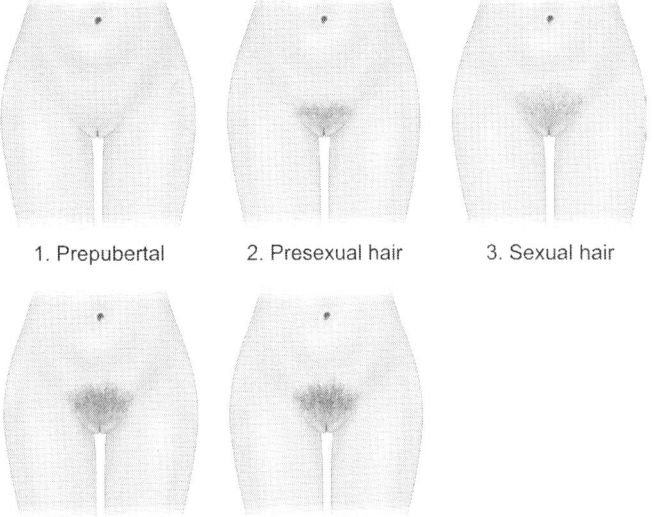

Fig. 1.1: Stages of adrenarche.

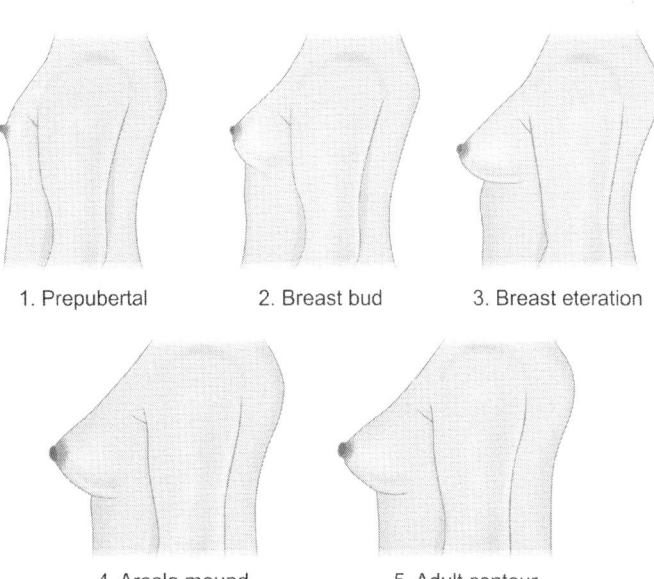

Fig. 1.2: Stages of thelarche.

- Vagina—epithelium becomes stratified. Cells are rich in glycogen due to estrogen and pH becomes acidic (pH—5) due to conversion of glycogen to lactic acid by Doderlein's bacilli.
- Vulva—increase in size of mons pubis and labia minora.

DELAYED PUBERTY OR INTERRUPTED PUBERTY

It is defined as failure of development of any secondary sexual characteristics by 13 years of age and nonachievement of menarche by 15-year of age and 95th percentile considered is 14.5-year which means 95% of children of that sex and culture have begun sexual maturation by that time.

Etiology of Delayed or Interrupted Puberty

- Structural abnormalities of genital outflow tract:
    - Müllerian dysgenesis (Mayer-Rokitansky-Kuster-Hauser syndrome).
    - Distal genital tract obstruction:
        - Imperforate hymen.
        - Transverse vaginal septum.
- Hypergonadotropic hypogonadism (FSH >30 mIU/mL):
    - Gonadal dysgenesis with stigmata of Turner syndrome.
    - Pure gonadal dysgenesis:
        - 46XX
        - 46XY
    - Early gonadal failure with apparent normal ovarian development.
- Hypogonadotropic hypogonadism (LH and FSH <10 mIU/mL):
    - Constitutional delay.
    - Isolated gonadotropin deficiency:
        - Associated with midline defects (Kallmann syndrome).
        - Independent of associated disorders.
        - Willi syndrome.
        - Laurence-Moon-Bardet-Biedl syndrome.
        - Other rare syndromes.
    - Associated with multiple hormone deficiencies.
    - Neoplasm of hypothalamic—pituitary area:
        - Craniopharyngiomas
        - Pituitary adenomas
        - Other.
    - Infiltrative processes (Langerhans cell—type histiocytosis).
    - After irradiation of CNS.
    - Chronic diseases with malnutrition.
    - Anorexia nervosa and related disorders.
    - Severe hypothalamic amenorrhea.

- Antidopaminergic and gonadotropin-releasing hormone—inhibiting drugs (especially psychotropic agents, opiates).
- Primary hypothyroidism.
- Cushing syndrome.
- Use of chemotherapeutic (especially alkylating agents).

Diagnosis

It is based on following parameters:
- History and meticulous physical examination are of prime importance with special emphasis on growth.
- *History includes:*
  - Assessment of patient's growth pattern.
  - Nutritional habits.
  - Intensity of exercise.
  - Any chronic illness.
  - Positive family history of constitutional delay.
  - Psychosocial perturbation.
  - Use of any medicine which can slow down pubertal growth.
  - No or anosmia.

Physical Examination

- Assessment of height, weight and arm span should be taken. If the arm span exceeds height by more than 5 cm, delayed epiphyseal closure secondary to hypogonadism is suspected. Height velocity must be determined for minimum six months and it should be charted on the one of available growth charts (Flowchart 1.3).
- Secondary sexual characteristics should be staged accordingly to Janner criteria also called sexual maturity rating (SMR). Presence of mature or immature secondary sexual characteristics and asynchronous development (breasts > pubic hair) should be carefully noted.
- Appearance of breast bud is the earliest sign of puberty evident in girls.
- In boys size of testis is measured by Prader over vidometer as it is the earliest sign of pubertal development. It corresponds to 2–3.1 cm in length and more than equal to 4 mL in volume.
- Symmetry of testis should be paid proper attention as many intersex disorders can present with asymmetrical gonadal development and defects in sexual maturation.

Imaging Modalities

- X-ray of non-dominant hand (usually left hand and wrist) for evaluation of bone age. It provides useful information about chronological age and skeletal maturation.

Flowchart 1.3: History and physical examination.

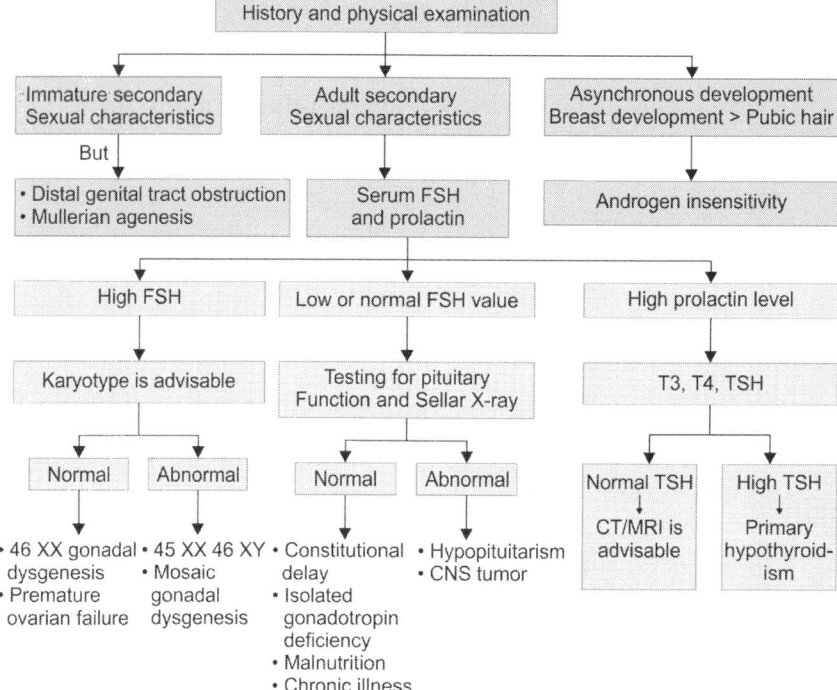

(FSH: follicle-stimulating hormone; T3: triiodothyronine; T4: thyroxine; TSH: thyroid-stimulating hormone; CT: computed tomography; MRI: magnetic resonance imaging; CNS: central nervous system).

- Ultrasonography (USG) test pelvis to confirm presence or absence of uterus and it is required when ovarian or testicular mass is detected on physical examination.
- Computed tomography (CT) or magnetic resonance imaging (MRI) scan is needed in the background of neurological symptoms or laboratory evacuation pointing towards hypothalamic or pituitary disease.

Biochemical or Laboratory Evaluations

- Preliminary investigation includes complete blood count, erythrocyte sedimentation rate (ESR), blood urea nitrogen (BUN), creatinine and liver function test.
- Hormonal test involves—serum LH, serum FSH, serum estradiol and serum testosterone which helps in differentiating between primary and secondary hypogonadism.
- Elevated serum prolactin levels suggests hyperprolactinomas which can cause "stalled" puberty and can result from prolactinomas or any hypothalamic or pituitary.

- Thyroid function test—elevated thyroid-stimulating hormone (TSH) suggests primary hypothyroidism which delays puberty by unknown mechanism.
- Assessment of adrenal androgens particularly DHEAS and sex steroids of adrenal origin helps to differentiate congenital GnRH deficiency from constitutional delay of puberty.
- Karyotype or comparative genomic hybridization (CGH) is recommended in every patient with primary hypogonadism to seek for Klinefelter syndrome in boys and Turner syndrome in girls.

Treatment

Treatment is targeted on three underlying etiology such as:
- Thyroid hormone replacement in primary hypothyroidism.
- Dopamine agonist treatment in cases of prolactinomas.
- Removal of craniopharyngiomas causes rapid sexual maturation in apt clinical scenario.
- The diagnostic dilemma between congenital GnRH deficiency and constitutional delay of puberty can be only unfolded with:
  - Subsequent vigilant observation, reassurance and psychological support for the patient and family.
  - Institution of gonadal steroids.
- Hormonal therapy for short period with testosterone for boys and estrogen for girls may be required to ameliorate unnecessary anxiety regarding delay and to relieve them from peer pressure under restricted scenario.
  - Exogenous estrogen for enhancing sexual maturation should be started in patients who was psychologically fit, at 12–13 years of age and after GH therapy was instituted for several years.
  - In girls estrogen therapy may be given orally or transdermally. Conjugated estrogen 0.3 mg daily or oral micromized estradiol 0.25 mg/day or transdermal estradiol 14 µg/day can be started in cases of hypogonadism. Cyclic progestin therapy with oral micronized progesterone 200 mg or medroxyprogesterone acetate 5–10 mg for 12–14 days every 1–2 month is added after 6–12 months of unopposed estrogen therapy or when breakthrough bleeding occurs.

PRECOCIOUS PUBERTY

Puberty is described as precocious when there is development of secondary sexual characteristics before the age of 8 years or menstruation occurring before 10 years of age. It implies that the limits are 2–2.5 standard deviation earlier than the mean age of onset of puberty.

Causes of Precocious Puberty

- *Central precocious puberty*: Dependent or central precocious puberty or true precocious puberty—is caused by early maturation of hypothalamic-pituitary-gonadal axis.
- *Peripheral precocious puberty*: Independent or peripheral precocious puberty—occurs due to secretion of sex steroids (estrogen and androgen) or human chorionic gonadotropin (hCG) independent of hypothalamic-pituitary gonadotropin stimulation.

Central Precocious Puberty

Patients have accelerated linear growth for age, advanced bone age and pubertal levels of LH and FSH.

Causes

- Idiopathic accounts for 80–90% of cases.
- *Central nervous system lesion*:
  - Hamartomas—most common type of CNS tumor to cause precocious puberty other are—astrocytoma, ependymomas, gliomas.
  - CNS irradiation—this precocious puberty is associated with growth hormone deficiency.
  - Others—infections, hydrocephalus, trauma, cyst.
- *Genetics*:
  - Specific gene mutations such as gain of function mutation in kisspeptin 1 gene (KISS 1).
  - Loss of function mutation in delta-like 1 homolog (DLK 1) gene.
- Previous excess sex steroid intake—patients treated with high level of exogenous hormonal therapy, e.g. congenital adrenal hyperplasia (CAH).
- Pituitary gonadotropin—secreting tumors.

Peripheral Precocious Puberty

It is caused due to excess secretion of sex hormones from gonads or adrenal glands or due to exogenous administration:
- Can be isosexual or contrasexual.
- Follicle-stimulating hormone and LH are suppressed and do not increase with GnRH stimulation.

Causes

- *Ovarian cysts:* It is three-most common cause of peripheral precocity.
- *Ovarian tumors:* Granulosa cell tumors, Sertoli cell, Leydig cell tumors.
- *Primary hypothyroidism:* Patients have early breast development, galactorrhea. Patient responds to thyroxine treatment.

Normal and Abnormal Puberty

- Exogenous sex steroids.
- *Adrenal pathology:* Androgen secreting tumors, congenital adrenal hyperplasia.
- *McCune-Albright syndrome:* It is defined as combination of peripheral precocious puberty, café-au-lait spots and fibrous dysplasia of bone.

Benign Pubertal Variants

This include:
- Isolated premature thelarche—most cases are idiopathic, they remit spontaneously and many do not progress:
    - Can be isolated unilateral or bilateral breast development.
    - Absence of other secondary sexual characteristic.
    - Normal height velocity for age.
    - Normal bone age.
- *Isolated premature adrenarche*: Appearance of pubic and/or axillary hair before 8 years of age along with serum DHEAS.
- *Isolated premature menarche*: It is very rare:
    - And consideration must be given to presence of infection, foreign body, abuse and trauma.
    - Patients have normal growth, development and fertility.

Diagnosis of Precocious Puberty

- To rule out: Tumors of CNS, ovary and adrenal glands.
- To determine the progress.
- To exclude causes such as foreign body, trauma, vaginitis, or genital tumors.

Physical Examination

- Height, weight, body mass index (BMI).
- Growth chart.
- Tanner staging (pubertal staging).
- Changes in external genitalia.
- Abdominal, pelvic, neurologic examination.
- Evidence of androgenization.
- Signs of hypothyroidism.

Laboratory Diagnose

- Bone age
- Head MRI
- Ultrasound abdomen and pelvis
- FSH, LH, hCG assays

- Thyroid function tests (TSH and free T4)
- Steroids (S. DHEAS, testosterone, estradiol progesterone, 17-OH progesterone)
- Inhibin levels
- GnRH testing.

When all signs of sexual precocity are present and basal or stimulated gonadotropin is in pubertal range (FSH >7.5 IU/L and LH >15 IU/L), pituitary secretion of gonadotropins is suspected:

- Any neurologic abnormality indicates CNS pathology.
- If examination and MRI are normal—idiopathic is the most likely diagnosis.
- If gonadotropins are suppressed along with increased estradiol—an ectopic source of hCG should be considered.
- Feminizing adrenal tumor should be suspected if there is elevated androgen with slight rise in serum estradiol and decreased gonadotropins.
- Accelerated growth and skeletal maturation along with sexual precocity in absence of virilization point towards ovarian tumor or cyst. FSH and LH are decreased but serum estradiol is elevated.
- Sexual precocity in presence of virilization indicates adrenal hyperplasia or a virilizing adrenal or ovarian tumor.
    - 21-OH (21-hydroxylase) deficient adrenal hyperplasia:
        - 17-OH progesterone
        - ↑ adrenal androgen.
    - 11-β-hydroxylase deficient adrenal hyperplasia:
        - S.11-deoxycortisol.
    - Adrenal tumor or a virilizing ovarian tumor:
        - Normal 21-hydroxylase
        - Normal 11-β-hydroxylase
        - DHEAS
        - Androstenedione.
- Development of breast, pubic hair and vaginal bleeding in a short child, with delayed bone age makes the diagnosis of primary hypothyroidism.

Treatment

Objectives

- To diagnose and treat intracranial disease.
- To arrest maturation until normal pubertal age.
- To diminish established precocious features.
- To maximize eventual adult height.
- To give psychological support or counseling.

- *Gonadotropin-releasing hormone agonist*:
    - Produces initial short-term flare followed by desensitization and down regulation of gonadotropins release thereby decreasing steroid production.
    - There is substantial regression of pubertal characteristic amenorrhea, and decrease in growth velocity.
    - Final bone height in increased due to delayed epiphyseal fusion.
    - Dose of GnRH agonist is monitored by assessing estradiol levels and aim is to keep estradiol less than 10 pg/mL.
    - Treatment is continued till epiphyses are fused or appropriate pubertal and chronologic ages are matched.
    - This is effective for central sexual precocity and not for peripheral cause such as CAH, McCune-Albright syndrome.
- Treatment for peripheral sexual precocity is to suppress gonadal steroidogenesis. The main drugs available are:
    - Acetate is used in depot form to suppress LH.
    - Aromatase inhibitors can also be used.
- Treatment of precocious puberty is directed towards the underlying disorder. If specific etiology is identified, then treatment must be individualized according to the diagnosis:
    - Surgical excision is the treatment of choice in case of ovarian or adnexal tumor.
    - Primary hypothyroidism can be successfully treated with thyroxine replacement.
    - In adrenal hyperplasia appropriate doses of glucocorticoids and/or mineralocorticoids can prevent further progression of pubertal development.

CONCLUSION

- Clinically delayed puberty is defined as an age at which 95% of children of that sex and culture have not attained menarche by 15 years of age or absence of development of secondary sexual characteristics by 13 years of age.
- History and physical examination are of utmost valve as tury help in establishing extent of pubertal development whether puberty has initiated but then stalled or its complete absence.
- High levels of LH and FSH indicate primary hypogonadism, whereas low to normal levels of LH and FSH indicate secondary hypogonadism.
- Differentiation of constitutional delay of puberty from other causes of delayed puberty is difficult and serial observations with watchful waiting are often required.
- Treatment should always be directed at underlying etiology.

- Physical examination involves␣anner staging of pubertal developmental and management, weight and testicular size evaluation. Height velocity should be assessed over six months and charted over growth charts available.
- Serum LH and FSH, Prolactin, TSH and free T4 values forms important component of laboratory evaluation.
- Short-term hormonal therapy should always be given after 12–13 years of age with several years of GH therapy under restricted window.
- Precocious puberty is early onset of menarche, i.e. before 10 years of age
- Causes can be central or peripheral.
- Clinical and laboratory evaluation should be done to find the underlying cause.
- Gonadotropin-releasing hormone agonists, medroxyprogesterone acetate and aromatase inhibitors glucocorticoids and mineralocorticoids can be used for the treatment. Surgical options may be used for mass lesions.

SUGGESTED READING

1. Hoffman BL, Schorge JO, Bradshaw KD, et al. Williams Gynecology, 3rd edition. New York: McGraw-Hill Education/Medical; 2016.
2. Jennifer Harrington. Definition, etiology, and evaluation of precocious puberty. https://www.uptodate.com/contents/definition-etiology-and-evaluation-of-precocious-puberty.
3. Padubidri VG, Daftary S. Shaw's Textbook of Gynecology, 16th edition. Gurugram: Elsevier India; 2014.

CHAPTER 2

Menopause: Physiology and Symptomatology

Mala Srivastava, Mamta Dagar

DEFINITION

The diagnosis of menopause is a retrospective diagnosis. The menopause is defined as the final menstrual cycle followed by one year of amenorrhea.

The word menopause is a Greek word "menos" (month) and "pausis" (i.e. stoppage or cessation). But, the physiological changes which cause the last menstrual period begin many years prior to menopause.

A dynamic neuroendocrine changes occurring during menopause is due to gradual reduction in the ovarian reserve. These phases of changes are known as "the climacteric." The word climacteric is a Greek letter and it means climbing the ladder or going up to the menopause. This period may or may not present with difficult physical and psychological problems.

PREMATURE OVARIAN FAILURE

If the menopause occurs before 40 years it is called premature ovarian failure. If the menopause occurs before 45 years it is known as an early menopause. The reasons for premature ovarian failure and early menopause include:
- Genetic cause, e.g. fragile X and Turner's syndrome.
- Idiopathic.
- Iatrogenic, e.g. girls who survive malignancies in younger age group by virtue of advanced treatment with advanced surgical techniques, radiotherapy and chemotherapy may have premature ovarian failure or early menopause.

PHYSIOLOGY

Menopause results when ovaries become less sensitive to the stimulation by gonadotropin-releasing hormone (GnRH) and is associated to follicular atresia. The oocytes become atretic throughout the lifetime of a woman. As a result there is a drop in follicular quality and the quantity as the women ages. Hence, the length of menstrual cycle varies during the climacteric period and is due to decreasing size of follicular cohort.

Anovulatory cycles and irregular cycles become common. There is a great variation in the production of GnRH, estrogen and progesterone, besides the sensitivity to these hormones also varies. Subsequently, there is a last menstrual period, and permanent amenorrhea occurs.

The irregularity of the hormone is not responsible for all abnormal bleeding which occurs during menopausal transition. So, the other pathologies, fibroids of uterus, polyps of the uterus and cervix, endometrial hyperplasia, or carcinoma of endometrium must be excluded either by endometrial biopsy or by dilatation and curettage (D & C). The histopathological diagnosis may confirm that irregular periods during climacteric may be due to hormonal irregularities.

The women in their 5th decade feels secure and they think that they cannot become pregnant, as they are nearing menopause. Though capacity to become pregnant decreases, yet pregnancy can occur in women aged between 40 years and 44 years. That means these women needs contraception.

The most common change during the menopausal transition is a shorter menstrual cycle (i.e. 25 days) among women with no pelvic pathology and who are ovulating.

The number of functional follicles, stimulated by follicle-stimulating hormone (FSH) during the early phase of the menstrual cycle, has fallen in number. So lesser number of oocytes is recruited, as a result the proliferative phase is shortened in these women. But, after the ovulation has occurred, secretory phase is static at 14 days.

As the time passes GnRH stimulation fails to recruit follicles and gradually FSH and luteinizing hormone (LH) levels starts rising. The raised FSH and LH level causes stimulation of the stroma of the ovary, and there is a rise in levels of estrone and a fall in estradiol levels. The inhibin—a hormone secreted by the ovary also drop during menopausal transition.

While there is the menopausal transition and there is a fall in the levels of functioning follicles, the characteristic changes occurs is there is a fall in the blood estradiol levels. The blood estradiol levels rapidly falls beginning two years before the menopause and plateaus about two years after the menopause. After menopause, there are no follicles, so the major part of estrogen in postmenopausal women is derived from androstenedione secreted by the ovarian stroma or from adrenals. This androstenedione from adrenal and ovarian stroma is later converted by aromatization to estrone, which is the estrogen of the menopausal ladies.

During the menopausal transition the levels of the serum testosterone does not alter much, and dehydroepiandrosterone sulfate (DHEAS) levels do change with age. Again during menopausal transition there are higher levels of total cholesterol, low-density lipoprotein (LDL), and apolipoprotein B (apoB) levels, together with lower levels of high-density lipoprotein (HDL).

After menopause when ovulation stops, the ovarian stroma produces estrogen in the peripheral tissue. The estrogen is also produced in the other sites, e.g. adipose tissue, muscle, liver, bone, bone marrow, fibroblasts, and hair roots, and there is no progesterone produced by the corpus luteum and there is no ovulation. As a result, perimenopausal and menopausal ladies have undoubtedly exposure to unopposed estrogen for long periods. This effect of estrogens can cause endometrial hyperplasia, which is a precursor of endometrial cancer (CA). The estradiol (E2) levels falls markedly among menopausal women due to loss of antral follicles. The estrone produced by aromatization from androstenedione is the major estrogens in the menopausal women.

Since, estrogens are produced in the peripheral fatty tissue, it may seem that the obese ladies will have higher levels of estrogens, and hence they should have lesser menopausal symptoms especially the vasomotor symptoms. But, this is not true, and vasomotor symptoms can be equally frequent and troublesome in obese women as they are in their slimmer counterparts.

The rising level of serum FSH levels is a clinical indication that there is menopausal transition. The level of FSH rises more than the levels of LH. A minor elevation or borderline increases in the FSH level during the menopausal transition is not a reliable indicator for the diagnosis of menopause. As, there is an elevated levels of GnRH and a lot of variation in the levels of FSH and LH.

To diagnose whether the woman is having menopausal transition or not, the levels of FSH and LH are repeated at 2–3 monthly intervals. The women with raised levels of FSH though not yet menopausal, are at risk for getting pregnant. So the contraception should be judiciously used in these women until they attain menopause.

LIPIDS AND LIPOPROTEINS

The estrogens affect the cardiovascular system. The protective effect of estrogens in women of reproductive age group is caused by high-levels of HDL and low-levels of LDL. The nitric oxide also causes vasodilatation and increase in the myocardial blood flow. After menopause women have raised levels of cholesterol, triglyceride and LDL levels, low-levels of HDL and an elevation of the insulin resistance.

CENTRAL NERVOUS SYSTEM

The estrogens affect the vessels of the central nervous system (CNS) and promote neuronal growth. They also improve cerebral blood flow and cognition in women lesser than 60 years. There is no benefit for dementia in older women even after giving estrogens. But in this age group there may be presence of the prothrombotic effect of estrogen, and there may be an increased risk of hormone replacement therapy (HRT) among these women.

PREDICTION OF MENOPAUSE

The 2nd day FSH levels are measured for assessment of reducing reserve in ovary and a value of more than 10 IU/L suggests lower ovarian reserve and more than 40 IU/L is considered diagnostic of menopause. But, sometimes these levels may mislead; as the levels varies depending on the timing of the sample and may vary in different cycles and is dependent on the ovarian activity as well. The anti-Müllerian hormone (AMH) levels are better predictor of ovarian reserve as it is produced by the ovarian follicles. Besides, the measurement of antral follicles by ultrasonography is also a good predictor of an ovarian reserve. The levels of AMH does not vary with the day of cycle and its prediction of ovarian reserve lasts for up to two years from when the sample was measured.

EVALUATION OF THE WOMEN

The menopause is diagnosed by:
- The history of the symptoms like hot flushes and night sweats.
- The variable periods of amenorrhea.
- The assessment of levels of E2, FSH, and LH among ladies with history of hot flushes is not necessary as they do not change the clinical management.
- But, in the younger woman or the one with surgical menopause, measurement of FSH, E2 and LH are useful, in planning the clinical management. The repeated levels FSH above or equal to 15 IU/L can be regarded as menopausal transition.
- Women who have been diagnosed as a case of spontaneous premature ovarian failure should be screened for autoantibody, karyotype and fragile X genetic analysis, in addition to hormonal level measurements.
- Once the diagnosis of menopausal transition has been made, investigations mean regular annual screening and this is applicable to all middle-aged women.
- The annual gynecological screening means measurement of weight, BP and Pap smear or liquid-based cytology (LBC).
- The levels of lipid profile should be measured in ladies with high BMI with high risk for cardiovascular disease (CVD).
- If women on hormone therapy (HT) and still having symptoms of hot flushes, then it is advisable to do hormone levels, so that the dose can be adjusted.
- Women should check their breasts and perineum at regular intervals, and clinical breast examination with gynecological check-up should be done annually.

- Mammography should be performed every two years unless any high-risk factor demands more frequent examinations.
- If a woman takes HT beyond 70 years, mammographic screening should continue till such time of HT intake.
- Among women 45 years and above, screening is by LBC, mammography and ultrasound of the pelvis preferably transvaginal scan (TVS) before commencing HT to have the baseline investigations of the patients.
- If the woman has no abnormal uterine bleeding then endometrial biopsy (EB) need not be done before starting HT.

The dual-energy X-ray absorptiometry (DEXA) of lumbar spine and hip is used for diagnosis of osteoporosis. But the biochemical markers of bone formation and bone absorption are better used to analyze the changes which occur before any changes in the bone density. The DEXAs should be done every two years. According to World Health Organization (WHO) the osteoporosis should be treated by considering the bone mineral density (BMD), the age and build of the woman.

Menopause Markers

The following are the laboratory marker which helps in diagnosis of menopause:
- The serum FSH is increased and E2 and inhibin levels fall during climacteric.
- If the woman is menstruating then the levels of FSH are seen higher than LH, and together are more than that seen during surge before ovulation.
- High FSH levels marks ovarian failure, and the FSH rises before the LH rise; but the rising levels of LH is not essential for the diagnosis of menopause.
- During menopause transition there is hardly any changes in thyroid function.

Endometrial Changes

- The histopathology of the endometrial may be from mildly proliferative to atrophic in nature among menopausal women.
- After menopause the secretory changes are not seen, because no ovulation is occurring and so no corpus luteum is formed and there is no production of progesterone.
- The histopathological evidence of endometrial hyperplasia reflects excess of estrogen.
- Endometrial hyperplasia can also be screened by TVS findings [i.e. endometrial thickness (ET) > 5 mm].

Menopause and Symptomatology

Menopause is the permanent stoppage of menses due to inability of the ovaries to produce hormones. It is recognized when a woman does not get periods for 12 months consequently without any other cause. The *perimenopause* includes the periods beginning with the onset of first symptom of menopause, e.g. vasomotor symptoms, menstrual irregularity, and ends 12 months after the last menstrual period, while *climacteric* is the variable period before and after menopause.

Ovarian Function

The menopause is due to decline in the function of the ovary and may occur early in smokers than in nonsmokers. Usually the menopausal age is predetermined in intrauterine phase with intrauterine growth restriction and low weight gain in early childhood leads to an early menopause. The women with Down's syndrome may also have an early menopause.

The ovarian reserve of germ cells is limited. The maximum number of ovarian follicle may be 7 million during 20 weeks in utero. Thereafter there is a gradual reduction in their number until the number of oocytes gets exhausted may be by 51 years of age on an average. As the women ages there is lesser response of gonadotropins on the ovary, and this may occur actually few years before menopause. There is gradual increase in circulating levels of FSH and later LH, decline in estradiol and inhibin levels during menopausal transition. FSH level more than 30 IU/L is considered diagnostic of menopause.

SEQUELAE OF OVARIAN FAILURE

Short-term

Short-term sequelae include development of hot flushes, mood swings, urogenital and sexual alterations. Due to variation in attitudes to the menopause different women have different perception of these symptoms. The menopausal symptoms are lesser in women of Japan, China and North America may be due to their cultural differences. Recent studies have shown that highly educated women and those women who indulge in regular exercises have lesser symptoms.

Vasomotor Symptoms

The vasomotor symptom includes hot flushes and night sweats. These symptoms are due to alteration of the sympathetic nervous system among these women. As hot flushes and night sweats can occur at any time and may disturb the sleep which leads to sleep deprivation, irritable behavior and alteration of short-term memory and concentration of these women.

Mood Disorders

Mood disorders are associated with irritable behavior, depressive or anxious nature and mood swings, lack of interest in the work and an attitude of lethargy with lack of energy. Various studies indicate the menopause is not associated with increased rates of depression however previous mood changes and affective disorders may be a risk factor for depression during this age group.

Urogenital Atrophy

The urogenital tract develops in close proximity, as both genital and urinary tract arise from the primitive urogenital sinus. Estrogen receptors are found in the female urinary bladder, urethra, the pelvic floor muscle and the vagina. The urogenital symptoms such as discomfort in the vaginal area, difficulty in passing urine, dyspareunia, recurrent urinary tract infection and incontinence may become regular symptoms in menopausal women. At least one of these urogenital symptoms is present among more than 50% of these women. The vaginal microenvironment changes with menopause, mostly as a result of fall in ovarian estradiol concentration. The vaginal mucosa is thinned out and studded with neutrophils. In postmenopausal women there is alteration in the vaginal colonization of bacteria. Now the vagina is colonized with fecal flora instead of *Lactobacilli*. The *Lactobacilli* protects against bacterial infection of vagina and urethral infection. So the protective effect of lactobacilli is gone and these women are more prone to repeated urinary tract infection.

Sexual Dysfunction

As the age increases there is decrease in libido in both men and women. But after menopause more than 43% of women will have decreased libido, lesser sexual arousal, dyspareunia and inability to achieve orgasm. The underlying reasons for female sexual dysfunction are multifactorial.

Long-term

The delayed consequences of menopause include osteoporosis, cardiovascular disease and connective tissue atrophy which affect the women's health in long-term.

Osteoporosis

World Health Organization defines osteoporosis as a condition characterized by lesser bone density and alteration of microarchitecture of bone tissue that leads to increased bone fragility and a high risk of fracture. There is 35% of risk of osteoporosis during the life time in postmenopausal women (Table 2.1).

Osteoporosis affects both men and women, but generally men have fewer fractures than women. There is an ethnic variability in risk of osteoporosis

Table 2.1: Risk factors for the development of osteoporosis.	
Gene factors	Family history of osteoporotic fractures among 1st degree relatives
Constitutional	Lesser body mass index (BMI)/anorexia nervosa If menopause was attained lesser than 45 years of age
Endocrine disease	Cushing's syndrome, hyperparathyroidism, hyperthyroidism, hypogonadism, type I diabetes
Drugs	Corticosteroids >75 mg prednisolone or equivalent daily, gonadotropin-releasing hormone (GnRH) analogues
Lifestyle	Smoking, excessive use of alcohol, low intake of calcium, excessive exercise leading to amenorrhea
Disease	Rheumatoid arthritis, neuromuscular diseases, chronic liver diseases, malabsorption syndromes, post-transplantation bone loss

with Caucasian lady having increased rate of fracture than those of Afro-Caribbean origin. It is unlikely that there is a single gene defect for osteoporosis, but several possible factors include vitamin D receptor, estrogen receptor and collagen.

Bone density increases during childhood and adolescence and peaks during the 3rd decade. After the menopause, the bone loss occurs at a higher pace, approximately 5% per year which decreases after 5 year to 1% per year. Whereas in the men the bone loss occurs at the rate of 1% per year. The development of osteoporosis depends on the peak bone density attained and subsequent bone loss.

Clinically osteoporosis manifests by evidence of wrist, hip and vertebral fractures.

Cardiovascular Disease

The cardiovascular diseases are manifested by stroke and myocardial infarction. CVD rarely cause death among women during their reproductive years but it is the most common cause of death beyond menopause especially after the age of 60. Even in the oldest group, CVD mortality does not match with that of men and it is much lesser than their male counterpart.

Connective Tissue Atrophy

Estrogens are the cause for skin elasticity, glow and tightness. As the estrogen levels fall there is also evidence of skin ageing. As a result there can be signs of skin ageing for example wrinkles, dry skin and loss of elasticity, atrophy, mottled pigmentation and scanty gray hair. The damage to the skin is not only due to biological ageing due to estrogen deficiency but also due to extrinsic damage especially ultraviolet radiation and pollution.

CONCLUSION

- 51 years is the average age of menopause.
- If a lady attain menopause before 40 years the diagnosis of premature ovarian failure (POF) is made.
- The climacteric means the time during menopausal transition.
- The menopause is a retrospective diagnosis if there is no period for one year when the last menstrual period has occurred one year earlier.
- Rising levels of FSH or LH and falling levels of AMH and inhibin may predict the onset of menopause.
- Menopausal symptoms can be hot flushes, mood swings, urogenital infection, and sexual dysfunctions.
- Long-term consequences of menopause are osteoporosis and cardiovascular diseases.
- Skin ageing and wrinkles are an integral part of estrogen deficiency.

SUGGESTED READING

1. Butler L, Santoro N. The reproductive endocrinology of the menopausal transition. Steroids. 2011;76(7):627-35.
2. Henshaw SK. Unintended pregnancy in the United States. Fam Plann Perspect. 1998;30(1):24-9.
3. Lenton EA, de Kretser DM, Woodward AJ, et al. Inhibin concentrations throughout the menstrual cycles of normal, infertile, and older women compared with those during spontaneous conception cycles. J Clin Endocrinol Metab. 1991;73(6):1180-90.
4. Santoro N, Brown JR, Adel T, et al. Characterization of reproductive hormonal dynamics in the perimenopause. J Clin Endocrinol Metab. 1996;81(4):1495-501.
5. Santoro N, Randolph JF Jr. Reproductive hormones and the menopause transition. Obstet Gynecol Clin North Am. 2011;38(3):455-66.

CHAPTER 3

Vaginal Discharge: Normal and Abnormal

Mala Srivastava

INTRODUCTION

The vaginal discharge is one of the most common complaints in Gynecology Outpatient Department (OPD). All clinicians should be able to distinguish normal vaginal discharge from abnormal vaginal discharge. This differentiation helps in proper treatment of the patients and prevents overtreatment.

Vaginal discharge is the mucus that keeps the vagina moist, clean and protects from infection. It is normal in most women and girls.

NORMAL VAGINAL DISCHARGE

- Does not have a strong or unpleasant smell
- Clear or white
- Thick and sticky
- Slippery and wet.

Vaginal Discharge

- Secretions from cervix and glands, e.g. sebaceous, Bartholin's and sweat.
- Squamous cells shed from vaginal epithelium.
- *Lactobacillus* and other aerobic and anaerobic bacteria.
- Some leukocytes, electrolytes, proteins and lactic acid.
- It also contains leukocyte protease inhibitor secreted by the vagina which protects vagina against inflammation and infection.

The pH of vagina is acidic varying between 4 and 4.5. Before puberty and after menopause the pH is alkaline and may reach up to 7. During postpartum period and after abortion the acidity of vagina is reduced and the pathogenic organisms are able to survive and many cause infections.

Nonpathogenic excessive vaginal discharge is seen during:
- Ovulation
- Sexual arousal
- Pregnancy

- Puberty
- Premenstrual phase of cycle.

NATURAL DEFENSE MECHANISM OF VAGINA
- Vaginal skin is tough and is stratified squamous epithelium devoid of glands.
- pH is between 4 and 4.5 and it acts against bacterial growth.
- *Lactobacilli* maintain the normal ecosystem in vagina.

FLORA NORMALLY PRESENT IN VAGINA
- The normal flora of vagina in woman of reproductive age group has both aerobic and anaerobic bacteria.
- The anaerobes predominates the aerobics in the ratio of 10:1.

ORGANISMS NORMALLY PRESENT IN THE VAGINA

Aerobic Organisms

Gram-positive
- *Lactobacilli*
- *Staphylococcus aureus*
- *Staphylococcus epidermidis*
- *Diphtheroids*
- *Enterococcus faecalis*
- *Streptococcus* group
- *Actinomyces israelii.*

Gram-negative
- *Escherichia coli*
- *Klebsiella*
- *Proteus*
- *Enterobacter*
- *Pseudomonas* species.

Anaerobic Organisms

Gram-positive Cocci
- *Peptostreptococcus*
- *Clostridium.*

Gram-positive Bacilli
- *Lactobacilli*
- *Eubacterium*
- *Bifidobacterium.*

Gram-negative
- *Bacteroides*
- *Fusobacterium*.

Yeast
Candida albicans and other species.

Vaginal ecosystems are maintained by microorganisms which produce:
- Lactic acid
- Hydrogen peroxide
- Peptides such as acidosins and lactacin
- Leukocyte protease inhibitor.

CAUSES OF VAGINAL DISCHARGE

Prepubertal Girls
- Pinworm or *Enterobius vermicularis* infestation
- Sexual abuse leading to sexually transmitted disease (STD), e.g. *Neisseria gonorrhoeae* infection
- Fecal contamination of vagina
- Shigellosis
- Foreign body
- Streptococcal and staphylococcal infection.

Postmenopausal Age Group
- Atrophic vaginitis
- Forgotten intrauterine contraceptive devices (IUCDs) or vaginal pessaries
- Cervical polyps-cervical malignancy
- Endometrial carcinoma
- Fallopian tube carcinoma
- Vaginal and vulvar cancer.

In the reproductive age group, vaginal discharge is one of the frequent complaints with prevalence of 30% in OPD patients.

ABNORMAL VAGINAL DISCHARGE

Causes of Abnormal Vaginal Discharge in Reproductive Age Group

Infective Pathology
- Bacterial vaginosis
- Vaginal candidiasis
- Trichomoniasis

- Chlamydia
- Gonococcal infection
- Primary syphilis
- Viral warts.

Noninfective Pathology
- Cervical ectropion
- Cervical polyp
- Intrauterine contraceptive device
- Endometrial polyp
- Cervical cancer
- Endometrial cancer.

Evaluation

The vaginal discharge is caused by bacterial vaginosis, *Candida* infection and *Trichomonas* infection. About 7-70% of women with complaints of vaginal discharge will have no definitive diagnosis. During evaluation, the history regarding previous vaginal infections and previous treatment has to be noted. A complete menstrual and sexual history has to be recorded. The sexual history includes questions regarding age at first coitus, date of last sexual activity, number of partners, gender of those partners, use of condom or barrier protection, method of birth control, prior STD history, and type of sexual activity—anal, oral, or vaginal.

Examinations

- *General physical examination* to assess the ill health or poor nutrition.
- *Per abdomen examination* to rule out any lump or tenderness.
- *Local examination to assess the discharge:*
  - If the discharge smells fishy then there is chance of bacterial vaginosis.
  - If the discharge is thick and white-like cottage cheese then there is possibility of candidiasis.
  - If the discharge is green, yellow or frothy, the possible cause is trichomoniasis.
  - If the discharge is with pelvic pain then there is chance of chlamydia or gonorrhea infection.
- *Per speculum examination* to assess the vagina, cervix and look for any local cause for vaginal discharge.
- *Per vaginum examination* to assess the size of uterus, any adnexal mass and to rule out any other pathology.

Specific Investigations
- pH of vaginal discharge
- Whiff test
- Wet smear
- Potassium hydroxide (KOH) smear
- Gram staining
- Culture
- Endocervical smear
- Stool examination
- Urine sediments
- Immunological tests, e.g. trichomonal, candida infections and viral antigens of herpes simplex virus (HSV) done by enzyme-linked immunosorbent assay (ELISA)
- Molecular testing
- Liquid-based cytology (LBC) or conventional pap smear
- Imaging techniques: Ultrasonography for pyometra or tubo-ovarian masses and endometrial thickness.

First, a saline preparation can be inspected. A "KOH-prep" contains a swab-collected sample of discharge mixed with several drops of 10% KOH and then inspected under microscope.

BACTERIAL VAGINOSIS

The bacterial vaginosis is a condition that reflects abnormal vaginal flora. Due to various factors the symbiotic relationship of the vaginal flora shifts and there is predominance of anaerobic species, e.g. *Gardnerella vaginalis, Ureaplasma urealyticum, Mobilincus, Mycoplasma* and *Prevotella*. Patients with bacterial vaginosis have remarkable absence or reduction of the normal vaginal flora, e.g. *Lactobacillus* species (Fig. 3.1).

Risk Factors
- Douching of vagina
- Smoking
- Having sex while menstruating
- Use of intrauterine contraceptive device (IUCD)
- Sex at an early age
- Multiple partners.

There is presence of a nonirritating, malodorous vaginal discharge. The clinical criteria used to diagnose the conditions may have following characteristics:
- Saline preparation of vaginal secretion using microscope
- Whiff test

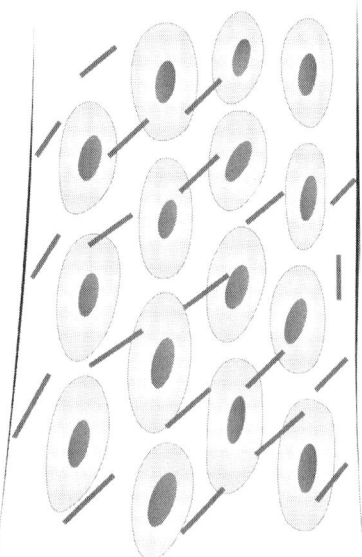

Fig. 3.1: Normal mature vaginal cells with *Lactobacillus*.

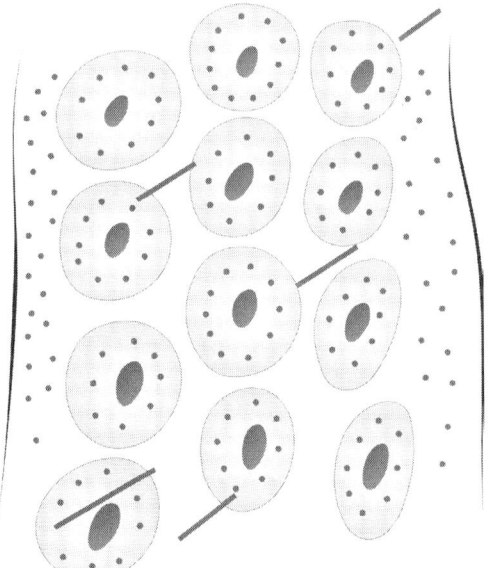

Fig. 3.2: Clue cells with very few *Lactobacillus*.

- Evaluating vaginal pH
- Presence of clue cells (Fig. 3.2).

The presence of clue cells and whiff test result though the patient is without symptoms. The pH of vagina in bacterial vaginosis is usually more than 4.5.

Three types of bacterial morphology are identified on staining:
1. *Lactobacillus*
2. *Gardnerella vaginalis or Bacteroides*
3. *Mobiluncus.*

Treatment

The treatment recommendation is given in Boxes 3.1 and 3.2.

FUNGAL INFECTION

Candida infection is seen more frequently in warm climates and in obese women. Besides, immunocompromised patients on steroids, diabetes, pregnancy, the recent broad-spectrum antibiotic are prone to fungal infections (Fig. 3.3).

With candidiasis infection, there are complaints of pruritus, pain lower abdomen, vulvar erythema, and edema with excoriations. The vaginal discharge may be white cheese-like. Vaginal pH is less than 4.5. The vaginal

---

Box 3.1: Treatment of bacterial vaginosis.

- Tab Metronidazole 500 mg two times a day × 7 days
- Metronidazole gel 0.75%, vaginally at bed time × 5 days
  OR
- Clindamycin cream 2% (5 g), vaginally at night × 7 days

Box 3.2: Other treatment regimen of bacterial vaginosis.

- Tab tinidazole 2 g daily × 2 days
- Tab tinidazole 1 g daily × 5 days
- Tab clindamycin 300 mg twice daily × 7 days
- Clindamycin vaginal passery 100 mg at bedtime × 3 days

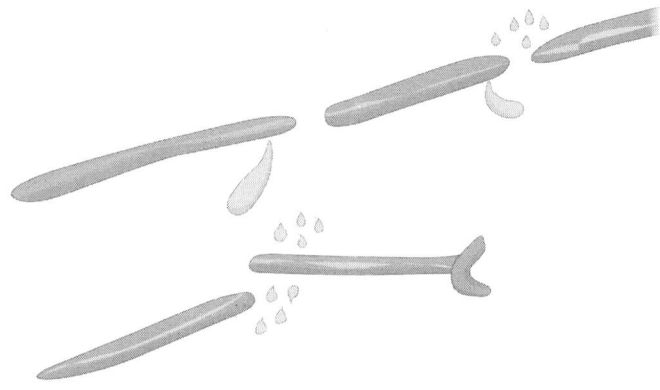

Fig. 3.3: *Candida* with budding.

> **Box 3.3:** Treatment regimen of fungal infection.
> - 1% clotrimazole cream 5 g vaginally daily x 14 days
> - 2% clotrimazole cream 5 g vaginally daily x 3 days
> - 2% miconazole cream 5 g vaginally daily x 7 days
> - 4% miconazole cream 5 g vaginally daily x 3 days
> - Vaginal suppository of 100 mg miconazole daily x 7 days
> - Vaginal suppository of 200 mg miconazole x 3 days
> - Vaginal suppository of 1,200 mg miconazole x 1 day
> - Ointment tioconazole 6.5% 5 g vaginally x single application
>
> *Other intravaginal substances which can be used:*
> - Vaginal cream butoconazole 2% cream x single application
>   Vaginal cream terconazole 0.4% 5 g vaginally once daily x 7 days
> - Vaginal cream terconazole 0.8% 5 g vaginally once daily x 3 days
> - Vaginal suppository terconazole 80 mg, daily x 3 days
>
> *Oral Drug:* Oral tab fluconazole 150 mg only once

discharge examined by microscope with saline or with 10% KOH preparations shows candida.

Treatment

Recommendation is to use any of the treatment regimens is given in Box 3.3.

TRICHOMONIASIS

The *trichomonas* are mobile flagellated, anaerobic protozoa. Their shape is oval and is slightly larger than white blood cells (WBC).

The incubation period of *Trichomonas vaginalis* varies from few days to weeks (Fig. 3.4). The urethra, bladder, endocervix and vagina can be infected. The discharge is classically seen as thin and yellowish or greenish with foul smell. There can be symptoms of dysuria, dyspareunia and vulvar pruritus.

The vulva may look red, edematous as well as excoriated. The vagina may contain the classical discharge and the subepithelial hemorrhage or "strawberry spots" which can be seen on the vagina and the cervix. *Trichomonas* is diagnosed in vaginal discharge by microscopic examination.

Vaginal pH is more than normal. The sensitive diagnostic technique is to culture, in Diamond's media. The nucleic acid amplification tests (NAATs) for trichomonal DNA are sensitive and highly specific. OSOM *Trichomonas* Rapid Test can also be used. It is an immunochromatographic assay, and has 99% specificity and 88% sensitivity.

Treatment

Recommendation is to use any of the treatment regimen is given in Box 3.4.

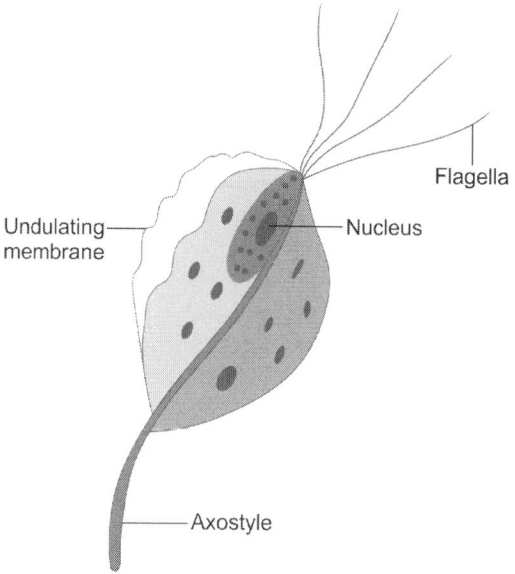

Fig. 3.4: *Trichomonas* vaginalis.

> **Box 3.4:** Treatment regimen of trichomoniasis.
> - Tab metronidazole 2 g, single dose
> - Tab tinidazole 2 g, single dose
>
> *Other alternate treatment can be*:
> * Tab metronidazole 500 mg two times a day x 7 days

NEISSERIA GONORRHOEAE

Usually *Neisseria gonorrhoeae* infections are asymptomatic.

Risk factors are:
- Young age
- Other STI
- History of infection with gonococci
- Multiple partners
- No use of contraception
- A profuse odorless, nonirritating and white-to-yellow vaginal discharge is usually present
- The *Gonococcus* may also infect the Bartholin's and the skene's glands and urethra. This infection can ascend upward and cause infection of the endometrium and the tubes.

Neisseria gonorrhoeae is a gram-negative *Coccobacillus* and causes columnar and infection of transitional epithelial cells. For gonococcal identification, NAATs are available.

*Recommendation is given in Box 3.5.

> **Box 3.5:** Recommendation for *Neisseria gonorrhoeae*.
> - Injection ceftriaxone 250 mg IM, only once
>   PLUS
> - Tab *azithromycin* 1 g only once

> **Box 3.6:** Recommendation for treatment of chlamydiasis.
> - Tab *azithromycin* 1 g, single dose
> - Tab *doxycycline* 100 mg two times a day x 7 days
>
> *Alternatively:*
> - Tab *erythromycin* 500 mg four times a day x 7 days
>   OR
> - Tab *erythromycin ethylsuccinate* 800 mg four times a day x 7 days
> - Tab *levofloxacin* 500 mg once daily x 7 days
> - Tab *ofloxacin* 300 mg twice a day x 7 days

CHLAMYDIASIS

Chlamydiasis is the 2nd most common sexually transmitted disease. Many infected women are asymptomatic. In women less than 25 years who are sexually active can have chlamydia infection and should be investigated annually.

This chlamydia infection is host cell-dependent for survival. It infects columnar epithelium and symptoms include mucopurulent discharge especially from endocervix.

To diagnose, culture with NAAT and ELISA are used.

Recommendation for treatment is given in Box 3.6.

SUMMARY OF CHARACTERISTICS OF COMMON VAGINAL INFECTIONS (TABLE 3.1)

Vaginal Discharge

- Normal vaginal discharge is not associated with foul smell or pruritus.
- Abnormal vaginal discharge may be associated with foul smell and abdominal pain.

Common Causes of Vaginal Discharge

- *Candidal infection:* Thick-curdy discharge associated with pruritus seen frequently in patients of diabetes or those patients on immunosuppressant drugs.
- *Treatment:* 2% clotrimazole cream 5 g vaginally daily x 3 days.

CONCLUSION

Table 3.1: Characteristics of common vaginal infections.

Types	Bacterial vaginosis	Candidal infection	Trichomonas infection	Chlamydial infection
Symptoms	Foul smell	Itching, and burning, together with discharge	Frothy discharge, foul smell, dysuria, pruritus, spotting per vaginum	No pruritus
Discharge	Thin, sticky, white or gray	Cottage cheese like white	Yellowish or greenish, sticky, frothy	Mucopurulent
KOH "Whiff test"	Present	Absent	May be present	Negative
Types	Bacterial vaginosis	Candidal infection	Trichomonas infection	Chlamydial infection
Vaginal pH	>4.5	<4.5	>4.5	<4.5
Diagnosis	"Clue cells," slight increase in WBCs in saline wet mount	Hyphae and buds (10% KOH solution wet mount) microscopy	Trichomonads seen moving (saline wet mount)	PCR and ELISA test

(ELISA: enzyme-linked immunosorbent assay; KOH: potassium hydroxide; PCR: polymerase chain reaction; WBCs: white blood cells).

Bacterial Vaginosis

- Thin profuse discharge diagnosed by wet smear, clue cells, KOH-examination, pH more than 4.5, positive whiff test and gram stain.
- *Treatment*: Clindamycin cream 2% (5 g) vaginally at night × 7 days.

Trichomonial Infection

- Profuse, green-frothy discharge associated with pruritus diagnosed by wet smear pH more than 4.5.
- *Treatment*: Tab tinidazole 2 g single dose.

SUGGESTED READING

1. Berek JS. Berek and Novak's Gynecology, 15th edition. Philadelphia: Lippincott Williams and Wilkins; 2011.
2. Centers for Disease Control and Prevention. CDC Guidelines. Atlanta: CDC; 2015.
3. Hoffman BL, Schorge JO, Bradshaw KD, et al. Williams Gynecology, 3rd edition. New York: McGraw-Hill Education; 2016.

CHAPTER 4

Abnormal Uterine Bleeding

Chandra Mansukhani, Anurag Vashista, Rashmi Nigam

INTRODUCTION

Abnormal uterine bleeding (AUB) is defined as bleeding from uterine corpus that is abnormal in regularity, volume, frequency or duration in the absence of pregnancy.

It is a common gynecologic complaint that may affect females of all age groups.

INCIDENCE

Abnormal uterine bleeding affects 10–30% of reproductive aged women and up to 50% of perimenopausal women.

Factors that influence incidence are age and reproductive status.

ETIOLOGY

It mainly depends on the age group to which the woman belongs:

Childhood

- Bleeding prior to menarche should be investigated as abnormal finding.
- Vagina rather than the uterus is the most common source of bleeding.
- Vulvovaginitis is the most frequent cause but dermatologic conditions, neoplastic growths or trauma by accident, abuse or foreign body may also be reasons.
- In case of true uterine bleeding, precocious puberty, accidental exogenous hormone intake or ovarian neoplasms should be considered in these children.
- Adequate evaluation may warrant examination under anesthesia with or without vaginoscopy.

Adolescence

- Abnormal uterine bleeding mainly results from anovulation or coagulation defects as compared with older reproductive aged women.

- Importantly, sexually transmitted diseases and sexual abuse should not be ignored in this age group.

Reproductive Age

- The hypothalamic-pituitary axis matures by this age and anovulatory bleeding is encountered less frequently.
- The rates of bleeding related to pregnancy and sexually transmitted diseases rise.
- The incidence of leiomyomas and endometrial polyps also increase with age. Bleeding from these lesions becomes common in older women within this age group.

Perimenopause

- Abnormal uterine bleeding is responsible for 70% of all gynecologic visits in this age group.
- Anovulatory bleeding from hypothalamic-pituitary-ovarian dysfunction is a more common finding.
- With aging, risks of benign and malignant neoplastic growths also rise.

APPROACH TO ABNORMAL UTERINE BLEEDING

The systematic approach to AUB has become more simplified and easy after the International Federation of Gynecology and Obstetrics (FIGO) nomenclature of AUB in 2011—The PALM-COEIN approach which includes structural as well as functional causes.

Previously various terms were used in literature to define pattern of AUB. However, they were inconsistently defined and it was difficult to compare results of various studies.

As per FIGO nomenclature, AUB has become universally accepted and there is consistency in defining the condition amongst various bodies. This has simplified the approach to the management with considerable uniformity and comparing the results based on various studies that are conducted at different places.

Based on the etiologies of AUB, FIGO in 2011 introduced the PALM-COEIN nomenclature that included structural (PALM) and functional etiologies (COEIN).

The structural causes include:
- **P**-Polyp
- **A**-Adenomyosis
- **L**-Leiomyomas (submucosal and others)
- **M**-Malignancy.

These are detectable through various imaging modalities and/or histopathology.

The functional causes include:
- **C**-Coagulopathy
- **O**-Ovulatory dysfunction
- **E**-Endometrial
- **I**-Iatrogenic
- **N**-Not defined that includes DUB (dysfunctional uterine bleeding).

The approach to case of AUB can be divided as:

Evaluation: History and examination.

Investigations: Laboratory, imaging, histopathology.

Management: Correction of anemia and as per PALM-COEIN classification.

Evaluation

History and Examination

- A detailed menstrual history must be taken including age at menarche, last menstrual period date and methods of birth control. The timing of her bleeding, bleeding amount and associated symptoms should be determined. Length of menstrual cycle, regularity and amount of bleeding estimated by number of pads changed per day should be noted.
- Screening for coagulopathies must be done especially in premenarcheal and adolescent age group.

Positive screen for coagulopathies include:
- History of heavy bleeding starting at menarche.
- One of the following:
    - Bleeding during surgery.
    - Bleeding during dental procedure.
- At least two of the following:
    1. Bruising more than or equal to 1 episode/month.
    2. Epistaxis more than or equal to 1 episode/month.
    3. Frequent gum bleeding.
    4. Family history of bleeding symptoms.

Examination includes measuring height, weight and body mass index (BMI); assess pallor and examination of thyroid, breasts and look for acne. In case of hirsutism, Ferriman-Gallwey (FG) scoring should be assigned.

The importance of thorough per abdominal, per speculum and per vaginal examination cannot be stressed upon.

Investigations

- *Ultrasonography (USG):* It should be done in all cases of AUB assessing uterus, adnexa and endometrial thickness (ET). It can be omitted in females less than 40 years of age up to 6 months of medical treatment.
- *3D USG:* It can be used as noninvasive alternation to hysteroscopy in selected cases like intramyometrial lesions or for fibroid mapping.
- *Doppler USG:* It is of help in cases of suspected arteriovenous (AV) malformations and malignancy. It can also be used to differentiate between fibroid and adenomyosis.
- *Magnetic resonance imaging:* It is of use in cases to differentiate between fibroids and adenomyosis, mapping of fibroids while planning conservative surgery and prior to therapeutic embolization of fibroids.
- *Saline infusion sonohysterography (SIS):* It is used in cases of suspected intracavitary lesions when hysteroscopy is not available.
- *Hysteroscopy:* It allows for direct visualization of intracavitary lesions and facilitates directed biopsies. The indications of hysteroscopy include:
    - Intermenstrual spotting
    - Intracavitary lesions
    - Ambiguity between symptoms and histopathology
    - Thick endometrial thickness (ET) on transvaginal scan (TVS) but HPE is inadequate or atrophic. No response to medical management.
- *Endometrial sampling:* This is recommended in all cases of age more than 40 years and in cases of age less than 40 years with high risk factors like:
    - Irregular bleeding.
    - Obesity, hypertension, polycystic ovary syndrome (PCOS), diabetes.
    - Unopposed estrogen therapy.
    - Endometrial thickness more than 12 mm.
    - Family history of cancer (CA) ovary or breast or endometrium or colon or hereditary nonpolyposis colon cancer (HNPCC).
    - Tamoxifen therapy for hormone replacement therapy (HRT) or breast cancer.
    - Persistent AUB, unresponsive to medical treatment.
- *Endometrial aspiration (EA):* This is one preferable technique. Dilatation and curettage is not recommended. *Hysteroscopy-guided sampling* has advantage over EA in that it can determine location of focal lesions found on USG. It can also serve as diagnostic as well as therapeutic benefit in the same session.

Management

Management of AUB can be either medical or surgical as shown in the flow chart followed by the detailed discussion of various aspects of medical as well as surgical management (Flowcharts 4.1 and 4.2).

Abnormal Uterine Bleeding

Flowchart 4.1: Medical management of abnormal uterine bleeding.

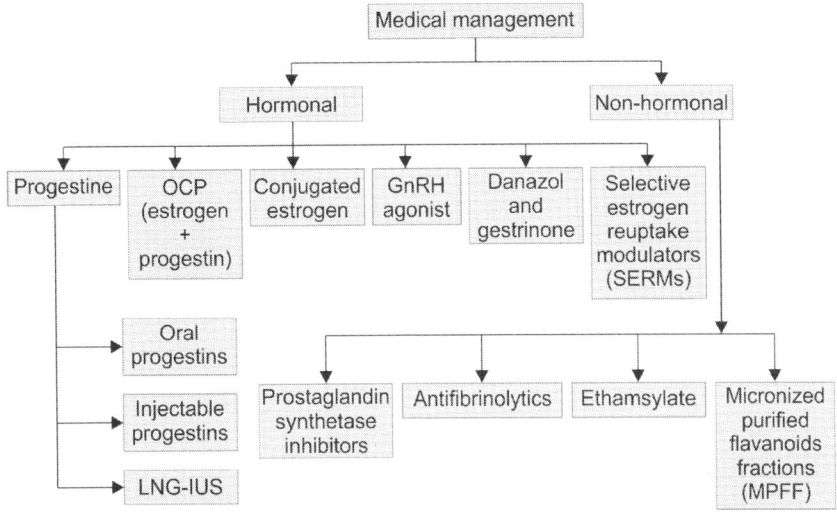

(GnRH: gonadotropin-releasing hormone; LNG-IUS: levonorgestrel-intrauterine system; OCP: oral contraceptive pill).

Flowchart 4.2: Surgical management of abnormal uterine bleeding.

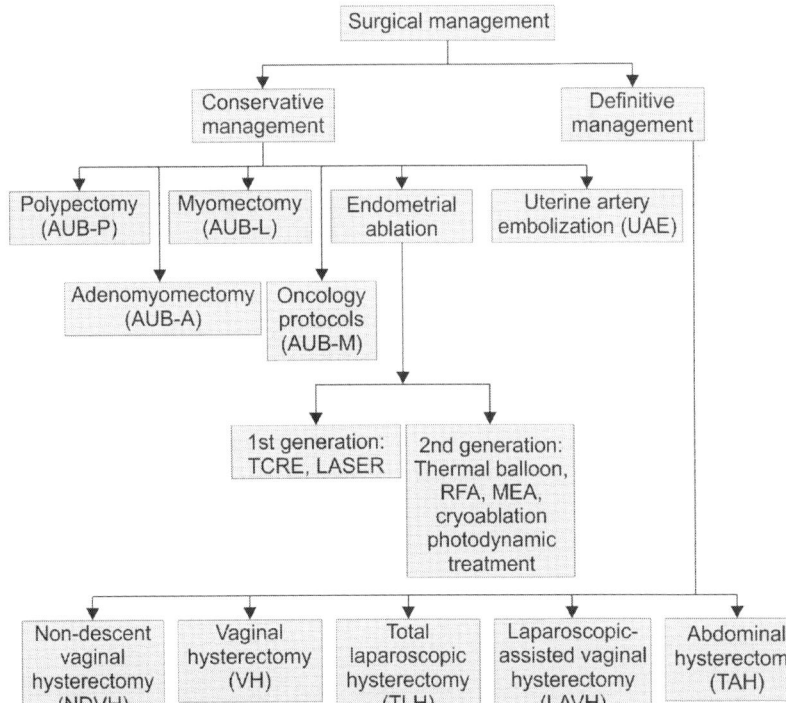

(AUB: abnormal uterine bleeding; LASER: light amplification by stimulated emission of radiation; MEA: microwave endometrial ablation; RFA: radiofrequency ablation; TCRE: transcervical resection of the endometrium).

Medical Management

Nonhormonal:
- Prostaglandin synthetase inhibitors (mefenamic acid):
    - It is usually the first-line of management for DUB in adolescent and reproductive age group. There is 30% reduction in menstrual blood loss and additional improvement in associated dysmenorrhea.
    - *Mode of action*: It inhibits cyclooxygenase (COX) enzyme and causes blockage of myometrial prostaglandin E2 (PGE-2) receptors.
    - *Regimen*: From the beginning of menstrual cycle, 500 mg thrice daily for 5 days.
    - Caution should be exercised in prescribing prostaglandin synthetase inhibitors, especially COX-2 inhibitors, to women with history of myocardial infarction, stroke and heart failure.
- *Antifibrinolytics (tranexamic acid)*:
    - These also constitute the first-line of management of AUB in adolescent and reproductive age group females, bringing about 50% reduction in menstrual blood loss. They are also useful in managing AUB related to IUCD (intrauterine contraceptive device).
    - *Mode of action*: They cause blockage of lysine-binding sites on plasminogen thereby reducing plasmin levels. This brings a reduction in fibrinolytic activity in endometrium. Thus the fibrin plug formed is not broken and this prevents and arrests the bleeding.
    - *Regimen*: Around 1–2 g per day in form of 650 mg thrice daily for 5 days starting from the beginning of menstrual cycle.
    - Antifibrinolytics have dose-dependent insignificant side effects like gastrointestinal (GI) upset. There is no alteration of coagulation parameters. However, they may not be effective or may have adverse reactions in women with history or risk of thromboembolism.
- *Ethamsylate*:
    - *Mode of action*: It maintains capillary integrity, has antihyaluronidase activity and inhibits prostaglandins. This causes platelet aggregation and adhesions resulting in formation of platelet plug.
    - *Regimen*: 500 mg QID starting from 5 days before anticipated onset of menstruation and continue for 10 days.
    - Ethamsylate is currently not approved by American College of Obstetricians and Gynecologists (ACOG) or Royal College of Obstetricians and Gynecologists (RCOG) and is still under trial for management of AUB.
- *Micronized purified flavonoid fractions (MPFF)*:
    - They cause increase in venous tone, lymphatic drainage and normalize capillary permeability.
    - Currently there is no evidence regarding their efficacy in treatment of AUB.

Hormonal
- *Progesterones*:
  - Progesterones bring a halt to endometrial growth and thus result in organized sloughing of the endometrium following withdrawal.
- *Oral progesterones*:
  - Two main progesterones used orally are norethisterone (NE) 5 mg and medroxyprogesterone acetate (MDPA) 10 mg.
  - *For acute heavy bleeding*: Superthreshold regimen is used to arrest an acute event of uncontrolled DUB. NE 5 mg is administered 4–6 times per day till bleeding stops and then twice daily for 2–3 weeks.
  - *For cyclical heavy menstrual bleeding*:
    - *Ovulatory cycles*: Ovulatory AUB is not usually due to progesterone deficiency but due to altered prostaglandin synthesis or hemostatic disruption. For ovulatory AUB, NE (5 mg) thrice daily or MDPA (10 mg) thrice daily is administered from 2nd to 25th day of each cycle.
    - *Anovulatory cycles*: Norethisterone (5 mg) twice or thrice daily or MDPA (10 mg) once daily is administered for 10 days. Withdrawal bleeding usually occurs 3–5 days following the 10 day course. It may also occur during or before the duration of course is over. This is followed by same dose taken from day 16 to day 25 following first day of withdrawal cycle for at least 3–6 cycles.
  - It is recommended to rule out endometrial carcinoma before starting progesterone therapy. Side effects of oral progesterones include mood alterations, weight gain, bloating, headache and atherogenic changes in lipid profile.
- *Injectable progesterone (Depo-Provera)*:
  - Depo-Provera (depot medroxyprogesterone acetate) 150 mg administered intramuscularly (IM) every 3 months is useful in managing AUB. There is additional benefit of contraception offered by the treatment. Prolonged use of Depo-Provera however, may cause a loss in bone mineral density and prolonged amenorrhea.
- *Levonorgestrel-intrauterine system (LNG-IUS; Mirena)*:
  - It effectively suppresses endometrial proliferation and lasts for 5 years from the time of insertion. There is decreased expulsion rate, added benefit of contraception and reduction in menstrual blood loss to an extent of 74–97%.
  - It can be used as first-line of management of AUB in reproductive and perimenopausal age group patients.
  - It is more effective in decreasing the blood loss as compared to mefenamic acid. The therapeutic effect of LNG-IUS is similar to endometrial ablation for up to 2 years of therapy. There is also

equal improvement in health status, quality of life and social well-being of women opting for LNG-IUS compared to those undergoing hysterectomy at 1 year and 2 years for management of AUB.
- *Contraindications to LNG-IUS are*:
  - Pregnancy (confirmed or suspected)
  - Uterine anomalies distorting the cavity (congenital or acquired)
  - Acute pelvic inflammatory disorder (PID) or history of acute PID
  - Postpartum endometritis or infected abortion in past 3 months
  - Abnormal pap smear or known or suspected uterine or cervical neoplasia
  - Genital bleeding of unknown etiology
  - Untreated acute vaginitis or cervicitis
  - Acute liver disease or benign or malignant hepatic tumor
  - Increased susceptibility to pelvic infection
  - Previously inserted IUCD that has not been removed
  - Known or suspected breast carcinoma
  - Previous ectopic gestation
  - Hypersensitivity to any component of mirena.
- *Combined oral contraceptive (COC) pills*:
  - Combined oral contraceptives bring about endometrial atrophy along with reduced endometrial fibrinolysis.
  - At least 30 µg of estrogen containing preparations are recommended.
  - Initially one pill every 8 hours is recommended till bleeding stops or reduced. The regimen continues for next 24 hours of stoppage of bleeding. The dose is then reduced to one pill every 12 hours for 3–7 days followed by one pill per day for next 21 days. This regimen is recommended for adolescent AUB and can also be used in perimenopausal age group patients.
  - There is additional benefit of contraception and reduction in associated dysmenorrhea.
  - Thus abnormal uterine bleeding associated with ovulatory dysfunction as defined by PALM-COEIN classification can be managed by nonhormonal and hormonal treatment with progesterones and COCs.
  - *Recommendations for abnormal uterine bleeding due to ovulatory dysfunction (AUB-O) management thus are*:
    - Both hormonal and nonhormonal therapies can be prescribed.
    - Combined oral contraceptives are first-line management for 6–12 months if fertility not desired.
    - Cyclic luteal phase progestins (D10-D14) are specific management.
    - If patient is not willing for COCs and wishes symptom free interval of at least 1 year, LNG-IUS is the choice of treatment.
    - Response is reassessed annually in such cases.

- Cyclic norethisterone for 21 days is used as initial therapy for acute episodes and should be continued for 3 months.
- Surgical treatment is not recommended unless AUB persists or is not responsive to medical therapy.
- *Conjugated estrogens (premarin)*:
  - In superthreshold doses, they stabilize endometrium and arrest bleeding. They also stimulate clotting at capillary level and promote vasoconstriction of spiral vessels.
  - They are used as hemostat for acute AUB episodes.
  - However, they are alone not recommended for treatment of AUB for long term as they can cause unopposed endometrial hyperplasia.
  - The recommended dose is 25 mg intravenously (IV) every 4 hours for up to 3 doses followed by 2.5 mg pill every 6 hours.
- *Selective estrogen receptor modulators (SERMs)*:
  - They are useful in case of perimenopausal DUB with hormonal deficiency. There is 60% reduction in menstrual blood loss.
  - The recommended dose is 60 mg twice daily for 12 weeks followed by 60 mg per week.
- *Gonadotropin-releasing hormone agonists (leuprolide)*:
  - They are helpful in short term to induce amenorrhea and allow women to rebuild their hemoglobin levels and red blood cell (RBC) mass. They are indicated in women awaiting natural menopause, surgery, young patients with medical disorders, anemia or immunosuppression.
- *Danazol and gestrinone*:
  - They cause hypoestrogenism and hyperandrogenism thus causing endometrial atrophy.
  - Danazol is given as 100–200 mg/day for 3–6 months and gestrinone is prescribed as 2.5 mg daily every 3–4 days.
  - They bring about a 60% reduction in blood loss. However, because of androgenic side effects, they are not used and are not recommended.
- *Abnormal uterine bleeding related to coagulopathy (AUB-C)*:
  - Around 13% of heavy menstrual bleeding (HMB) cases have systemic disorders of hemostasis.
  - The inherited ones include Von Willebrand disease (VWD), factor VIII, IX, XI deficiencies and platelet function defects.
  - Von Willebrand disease is commonest coagulation disorder presenting as HMB.
  - Nonhormonal treatment like tranexamic acid is used as primary line of management.
  - Hormonal therapy includes COCs and LNG-IUS.
  - In refractory cases, hematology consultation is needed.

- Specific factor replacement is to be done wherever possible.
- *Desmopressin is used as treatment for VWD*: When surgical intervention is indicated, appropriate preoperative, postoperative and intraoperative management is to be done with hematologist.

Surgical Management

- *Endometrial polyps and abnormal uterine bleeding (AUB-P):*
  - Polyps are localized tumors of columnar epithelium of endocervix or endometrial epithelium. They contain both glandular and stromal elements and are usually benign.
  - Hysteroscopic polypectomy is recommended in young women who wish to preserve fertility.
  - In women with multiple or recurrent polyps, the polyps should be sent for histopathology. If benign, LNG-IUS or endometrial ablation is the option. If it comes malignant, the treatment protocol is followed as per oncology.
- *Abnormal uterine bleeding associated with adenomyosis*:
  - Adenomyosis is estrogen dependent entity usually presenting as HMB and dysmenorrhea.
  - The cases must be individualized based on age, symptoms, associated pathology like leiomyomas, polyps or endometriosis and desire for fertility.
  - If fertility preservation is desired and immediate conception is not wished for:
    - Levonorgestrel-intrauterine system is first-line of treatment.
    - Gonadotropin-releasing hormone agonists with add back therapy are used for those unwilling for LNG-IUS.
    - Nonsteroidal anti-inflammatory drugs, combined pills and progestogens are used for symptomatic treatment.
    - Adenomyomectomy is reserved for selected cases.
  - If fertility preservation is not desired, LNG-IUS or GnRH agonist with add back therapy is used for medical management.
  - Hysterectomy is reserved for those not responding to medical treatment and not wishing for fertility preservation.
- *Abnormal uterine bleeding associated with leiomyomas (AUB-L)*:
  - Leiomyomas are the benign fibromuscular tumors of the myometrium.
  - They are classified from Type 0 to type 8 by FIGO based on their relation to endometrium.
  - The treatment is individualized based on age, parity, symptoms and desire for fertility or menstrual function preservation.
  - Usually, type 0–1 with size less than 4 cm is resorted to hysteroscopic myomectomy. Abdominal myomectomy is recommended for size greater than 4 cm.

- First generation ablation like transcervical resection of the endometrium (TCRE) are useful in selected cases undergoing hysteroscopic myomectomy but not desirous of pregnancy.
- Type 2-4 is usually managed medically with symptomatic management like tranexamic acid, COCs, nonsteroidal anti-inflammatory drugs (NSAIDs).
- If concurrent contraception is desired, LNG-IUS is the option.
- Myomectomy is reserved for the cases with associated infertility or failure of medical management.
- Hysterectomy is resorted to cases with age more than 40 years, symptomatic myomas and not desiring fertility.
- Levonorgestrel-intrauterine system can be given for type 3-4 myomas, selected type 2 myomas and contraindicated in type 0 and type 1.
- Selective progesterone receptor modulators (SPRMs) like ulipristal acetate or mifepristone are emerging as promising agents for the management.
- Gonadotropin-releasing hormone agonists with add back therapy is used as short term treatment for improving anemia, prior to myomectomy to reduce size and selected perimenopausal women to tide over menopause.
- Endometrial ablation is useful in cases of HMB with small uterine fibroids (<3 cm), uterus <10 weeks. Second generation ablative therapies should be used.
- *Abnormal uterine bleeding associated with malignancy (AUB-M):*
  - Follow-up of standard oncology protocol is recommended for AUB-M category women.
  - In case of hyperplasia with atypia, hysterectomy is the standard treatment.
  - If woman is young desiring fertility and has good compliance for regular follow-up, conservative treatment with high dose progesterones is an exceptional treatment.
  - In cases of hyperplasia without atypia, LNG-IUS is first-line therapy. Alternate option is oral progesterones. Endometrial aspiration should be repeated every 6 months.
  - Ablative therapy is not recommended because complete destruction is not ensured and histological follow-up is difficult.
- Conservative surgery (endometrial ablation).

Principles of Conservative Surgery

- To bring about destruction of endometrium in menorrhagia.
- Usually reserved for the cases following failure of medical management and before resorting to extirpative procedures.

- The endometrium has immense power to regenerate and the basal layer is responsible for regeneration.
- To bring about therapeutic Asherman's syndrome so as to arrest bleeding.
- The destruction should always occur from fundus to cornua to upper endocervical canal.
- The endomyometrial surface is irregular and must be destroyed.
- The burns can spill through oviducts and also affect serosa. Therefore caution is recommended and surgical expertise is desired to perform the procedure.

Choice of Patients

- Normal uterus with at least 3 months history of heavy menstrual flow.
- No intrauterine pathology including normal endometrial biopsy and pap smear.
- No evidence or suspicion of pregnancy, malignancy or infection.
- Endometrial carcinoma should be ruled out.
- Completed family is desirable.
- Normal endometrial cavity.

Food and Drug Administration (FDA) Guidelines for Conservative Procedures

Inclusion criteria:
- Uterine bleeding from benign causes.
- Failed medical management.
- Uterocervical length as measured by uterine sound should be less than 12 cm.

Exclusion criteria:
- Pelvic inflammatory disease
- Coagulopathy
- Abnormal pap smear
- Malignancy
- Pregnancy
- Previous ablation
- Previous uterine surgeries.

Preprocedure Counseling

- The main aim is to return the bleeding to normal levels or lesser. Amenorrhea is not the desired result.
- The woman may experience vaginal discharge which may be bloody during the first few days, serosanguineous after 1 week and profuse and watery thereafter.

- Around 10–20% of women may require hysterectomy.
- Appropriate contraception is recommended.

Pretreatment
- Postmenstrual is the preferred timing for the procedure.
- Pretreatment with GnRH agonist for 4-6 weeks is beneficial. However, optimum pretreatment method has not yet been determined.
- Nonsteroidal anti-inflammatory drugs are recommended 30–60 minutes before the procedure.
- Immediate prior suction or sharp curettage should be done.

Anesthesia
- Paracervical block or short general anesthesia (GA) is preferred for the procedure.
- The ablative procedures can be divided into two generations:
    - *1st generation*: Utilize hysteroscopy guidance. It includes neodymiumyttrium aluminum garnet (ND: YAG) and TCRE.
    - *2nd generation*: Nonhysteroscopy procedures. They utilize heat production for ablation from various energy sources like hot water, cryocautery, microwaves and radiofrequency waves. All these procedures can be done as office procedures under local anesthesia like paracervical block.

Endometrial laser interstitial thermal therapy (ELITT) is a newer ablative procedure that uses diode laser substitution. The main advantages are smaller unit and less expense involved. Clinical trials are ongoing and results are awaited for the efficacy of the procedure.

Definitive Surgery (Hysterectomy)
- It is the definite management but is now recommended as a last resort to the management of AUB and only after other procedures has failed. It is almost never done in case of adolescent AUB.
- The various routes by which hysterectomy can be done are open abdominal, vaginal and laparoscopy. The choice of route depends on surgeon's expertise and comfort.
- It is recommended to counsel the patient regarding various modes of management available and reach a decision making based on patient's desires and performance score.

Uterine Artery Embolization
- *Indications*:
    - AV malformation
    - Symptomatic fibroid
    - Preservation of uterus desirable but not fertility

- Poor surgical risks
- Severely anemic and requiring immediate intervention
- Symptomatic improvement is seen in 84% women in first 6 months, and 83% at 24 months. There is 40–70% reduction in fibroid volume. Around 15–20% cases would require other intervention like hysterectomy, myomectomy or repeat uterine artery embolization (UAE).

Magnetic Resonance Imaging-guided High-intensity Focused Ultrasound

It has emerged as newer technique and promises to be noninvasive outpatient basis procedure with no radiation exposure.

CONCLUSION

- Abnormal uterine bleeding is defined as bleeding from uterine corpus that is abnormal in regularity, volume, frequency or duration.
- It is a common gynecological problem affecting females of all age groups.
- Etiology mainly depends on the age group to which the woman belongs.
- Approach to AUB diagnosis and management is based on PALM-COEIN classification.
- A detailed history and examination helps in reaching the diagnosis.
- Ultrasound is main preliminary investigation needed in all cases of AUB.
- Magnetic resonance imaging, SIS and hysteroscopy are done depending on the need.
- Endometrial aspiration is done in carefully selected patients.
- Management may be medical or surgical.
- Antifibrinolytics, progesterones and COCs usually form the mainstay of medical management.
- Coagulopathy screening is required in cases of adolescent AUB and treated based on underlying cause.
- Surgical management depends on the type of lesion (polyp, adenomyosis, fibroid or malignancy).
- Endometrial ablation is reserved for carefully selected patients.
- Definitive surgical management is hysterectomy.
- Uterine artery embolization and HIFU are newer and promising modalities of treatment.

SUGGESTED READING

1. Berek JS. Berek and Novak's Gynecology, 15th edition. Philadelphia: Lippincott Williams and Wilkins; 2011.
2. Hoffman BL, Schorge JO, Bradshaw KD, et al. William Gynecology, 3rd edition. New York: McGraw-Hill Education; 2016.
3. UptoDate. (2017). Management of abnormal uterine bleeding. [Online] Available from https://www.uptodate.com/contents/management-of-abnormal-uterine-bleeding [Accessed September 2018].

Dysmenorrhea

Punita Bhardwaj

INTRODUCTION

Dysmenorrhea means difficult menstruation but the term is used to mean painful menstruation. It is of two types: (1) primary dysmenorrhea and (2) secondary dysmenorrhea according to the origin of pain. Primary dysmenorrhea is generally spasmodic and on first day of menses and secondary dysmenorrhea is congestive type and worst premenstrual and relieved by the start of menses.

DEFINITION

Dysmenorrhea is defined as pain associated with menses.

PREVALENCE

Dysmenorrhea is widely prevalent, more than 50% women suffer from this in their lifetime in reproductive period, 10% girls in their late teens are incapacitated for 2–3 days in each month.

TYPES

- *Primary dysmenorrhea*: Pain is of uterine origin and directly linked to menstrual origin but with no visible pathology in pelvis. It is caused by hypersecretion of prostaglandins and is common in young girls and has good prognosis.
- *Secondary dysmenorrhea*: Pain associated with uterine or pelvic pathology, e.g. endometriosis and adenomyosis, etc.
- *Membranous dysmenorrhea*: It is a rare form of dysmenorrhea with family incidence in which endometrium is shed off in large pieces or in a single piece of endometrium. It causes severe pain abdomen due to uterine contraction to pass this endometrium through the internal orifice (os).

ETIOLOGY

Primary Dysmenorrhea
Increased prostaglandins production with no pelvic pathology.

Secondary Dysmenorrhea
- *Endometriosis*: In endometriosis, endometrial glands and stroma are found outside the uterine cavity, especially at the pouch of Douglas, ovaries and pelvic viscera and parietal peritoneum (Fig. 5.1). Patient complains of severe dysmenorrhea and cyclic pelvic pain that starts 2 weeks prior to menses. Pain is localized in lower abdomen, back, and rectum.
- *Ovarian endometrioma or other tumors.*
- *Acute and chronic: pelvic inflammatory disease (PID)*: PID is polymicrobial infections with gram-negative and gram-positive bacteria. PID by *Neisseria gonorrhoeae* or chlamydia is manifested by acute onset of pelvic pain, with fever and purulent vaginal discharge. Subclinical cases of PID present with chronic pelvic pain and dysmenorrhea.
- *Broad ligament varicocele.*
- *In the uterus*: Adenomyosis—defined as presence of endometrial stroma and glands within the myometrium, at least one low power field from the basis of the endometrium (Figs. 5.2A and B). The average age of symptomatic women is usually older than 40 years.
- *Leiomyomas*: Uterine leiomyomas are uterine smooth muscle tumors. Patient may have discomfort when leiomyomas are present in broad ligament encroaching on adjacent bladder, rectum or supporting ligaments of the uterus. There is no association between degree of pain, fibroid volume and number (Fig. 5.3).

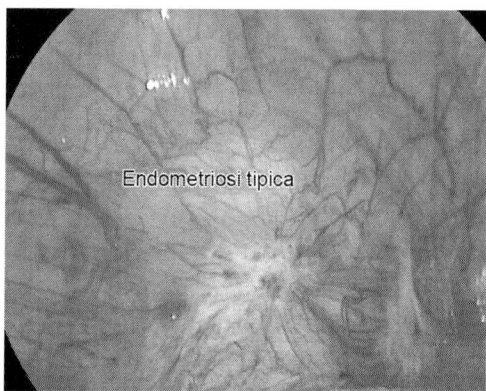

Fig. 5.1: Laparoscopic view of endometriotic lesion on the peritoneum.

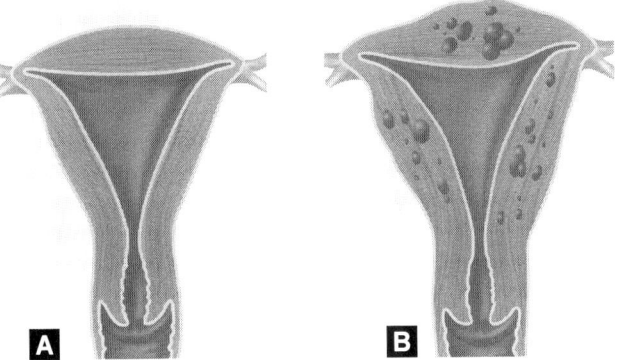

Figs. 5.2A and B: (A) Normal uterus; (B) Adenomyosis uteri.

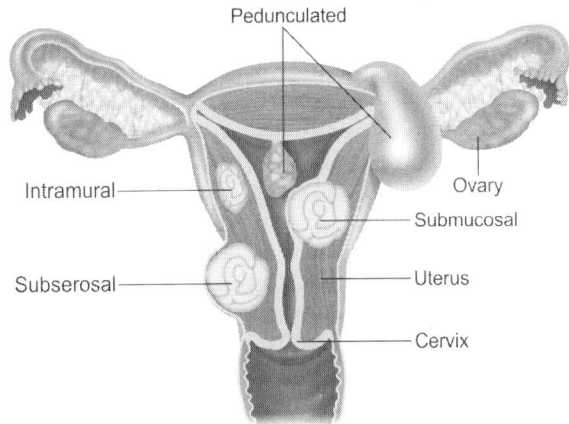

Fig. 5.3: Different sites of fibroid in the uterus.

- *Polyp*: Fibroid or endometrial polyp when pedunculated in endometrial cavity, the uterus contracts to expel it as a foreign body (Fig. 5.4). This pain is cramping in nature like a mini labor.
- *Intrauterine device.*
- *Intrauterine adhesions (Fig. 5.5).*
- *Cervical stenosis (Fig. 5.5).*
- *Imperforate hymen (Fig. 5.5).*
- *Bicornuate uterus:* Bicornuate uterus has indented fundus and two endometrial cavities (Fig. 5.6).
- *Septate uterus:* Septate uterus is normal externally but has two internal cavities (Fig. 5.7). This is developed due to a defect in canalization or

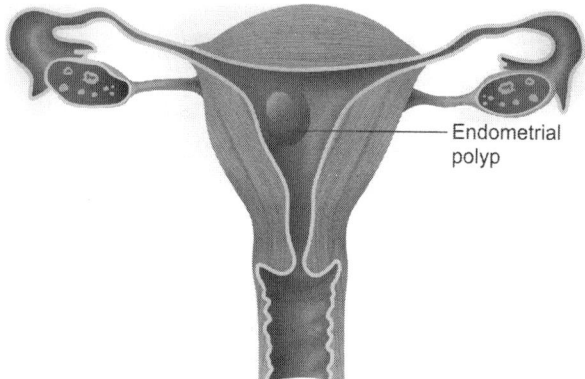

Fig. 5.4: Endometrial polyp in the uterus.

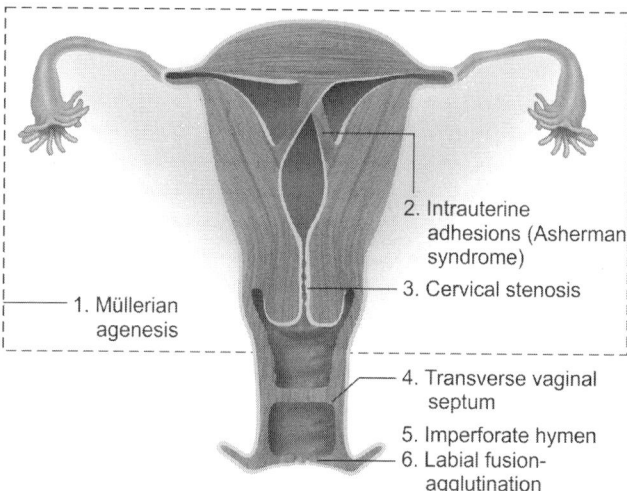

Fig. 5.5: Recanalization/abnormalities of uterus.

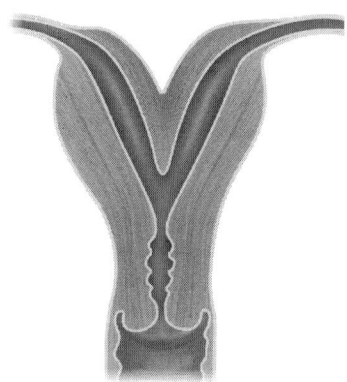

Fig. 5.6: Bicornuate uterus.

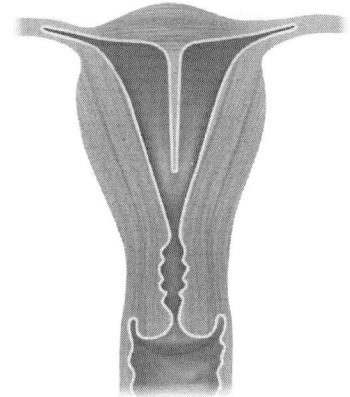

Fig. 5.7: Septate uterus.

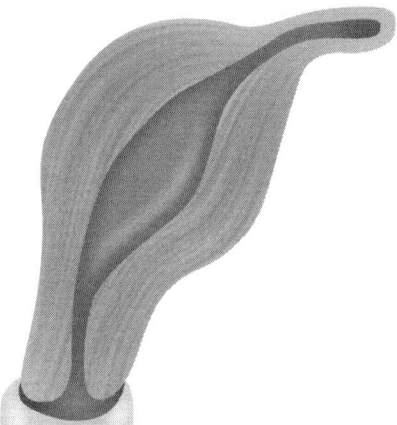

Fig. 5.8: Unicornuate uterus.

resorption of the midline septum between the two Müllerian ducts in intrauterine development. Partial and complete uterine septa are defined by the proximity of the septum to the internal os.
- *Uniconuate uterus (Fig. 5.8):* This is an asymmetric lateral fusion defect, one cavity normal, with a fallopian tube and cervix. This horn may or may not communicate with the uterus.
- *Uterus didelphous*: It occurs when the two Müllerian ducts fail to fuse. Uterus, cervix and vagina are separated from other half of it.
- *Rudimentary horns.*
- *Transverse vaginal septum.*

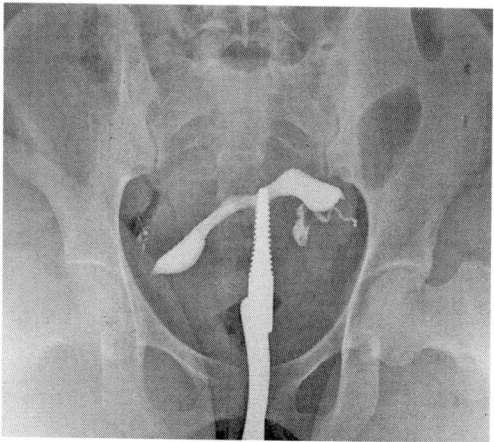

Fig. 5.9: Hysterosalpingogram.

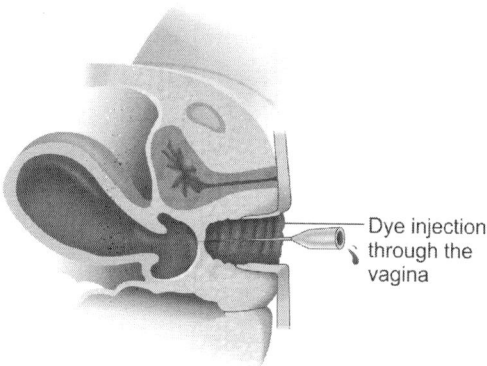

Fig. 5.10: Hysterosalpingography.

It is type of fusion defect in vagina may be longitudinal and transverse. When transverse may present as primary amenorrhea in complete variety and dysmenorrhea in incomplete or perforated transverse vaginal septum (Figs. 5.9 and 5.10).
- Post lower (uterine) segment cesarean section (LSCS) scared uterus.

SYMPTOMS

Pain starts few hours before the menstruation and continues for up to 2–3 days. Pain is in the form of cramps in lower abdomen radiating towards inner side of the thighs. Half of these cases have symptoms of nausea, vomiting, diarrhea, fatigue, irritability and dizziness. It contributes to the quality adjusted life years lost in this age group:

- During severe attack, patient may look drawn, pale and may sweat.
- Syncopal attacks are also seen in some patients.
- There may be diarrhea and rectal and bladder tenesmus.
- Severe dysmenorrhea appears only after 2–4 years of menarche.

Endometriosis
- Cyclical pelvic pain with menses may be associated with dysmenorrhea, dyspareunia, dysuria, dyschezia and subfertility.
- Pain is increasing for 2–3 days premenstrual but reaches its climax during or at the end of period.
- This pain persists for several days and only ceases completely after period is over.

Congestive Dysmenorrhea
- Reaches its height during 2 or 3 days preceding menstruation and is slowly relieved if congestion is reduced with the onset of menstruation.
- Backache may be the result of hormonal influences on spine and pelvis.

DIAGNOSIS
History
- Detailed history of pain, its associated features, duration and severity.
- Any chronic illness in past or operation performed.

Examination
- Abdominal examination for any obvious mass.
- Per speculum examination—to rule out pelvic inflammatory disease in sexually active patients.
- Pervaginal examination—to rule out any pelvic pathology in uterus and adnexa. Pouch of Douglas to be assessed for any nodularity as in case of endometriosis.
- Rectovaginal finding—fixed of retroverted uterus with reduced mobility, adnexal masses and uterosacral nodularity.

Investigations
- Complete blood count—for any inflammatory cause as pelvic inflammatory disease and urinary tract infection.
- Ultrasound—to rule out pelvic pathology, e.g. fibroid uterus, adenomyosis, polyp, forgotten intrauterine contraceptive device (IUCD), or congenital anomalies, etc.
- Computed tomography (CT) or magnetic resonance imaging (MRI) scan—for detailed anatomy of pathology diagnosed of ultrasound.
- Laparoscopy or hysteroscopy—according to clinical suspicion.

TREATMENT

Primary Dysmenorrhea

General Measures

- Bed rest during the first day or so of the period.
- Improvement in nutritional state and dietary changes including fruits, eggs and fish in diet.
- Applying heat, such as a hot water bottle, to the abdomen.
- Explanation regarding condition and reassurance.
- Regular exercise for 15 minutes daily, between and during menses with attention to overall physical fitness.
- Relaxation techniques.
- Palliative measures like laxatives and hot bath act by increasing blood supply and taking away ischemic elements.
- Psychotherapy.

Medical Management

- Nonhormonal:
  - Nonsteroidal anti-inflammatory drugs (NSAIDs): It is the mainstay of treatment.
  - Ibuprofen: 200–600 mg 6 hourly.
  - Mefenamic acid: 500 mg initially, then 250 mg 6 hourly.
  - Celecoxib: 400 mg initially, then 200 mg bd.
  - Naproxen: 450–550 mg initially, then followed by reduced dosage.
  - These drugs are used for 1–3 days from the onset of menses.

Hormones

- When prostaglandins inhibitors fail or are contraindicated.
- Cyclical hormone therapy for 6 months.
- Oral contraceptives (OCPs)—start from 5th to 25th day of cycle.

Surgical Treatment

- Only when pain is so sever as to incapacitating primary dysmenorrhea patients.
- Medical management has failed.
- Rarely indicated and hardly ever performed before the age of 18 years.
- Procedure followed:
  - Laparoscopy.
  - Dilatation of cervix.
  - Injection of anesthetic agent in pelvic plexus.
  - Presacral neurectomy.
  - Laparoscopic nerve ablation (LUNA).
  - Transcutaneous electrical nerve stimulation (TENS).

Secondary Dysmenorrhea
- Treatment according to uterine or pelvic pathology.
- Treatment—adenomyosis is excised for fertility preservation.
  - If family is complete or for recurrence of adenomyosis hysterectomy is done.
  - Leiomyomas prostaglandin synthetase inhibitors provide relief.
  - Endometriosis.
  - IUCD users.
  - In IUCD user alternative method of contraception should be used with removal of IUCD.
  - Rudimentary horns—if functional and symptomatic, best treatment is excision.
  - Reconstructive operation for malformed uterus.

Membranous Dysmenorrhea
- Pathogenesis is obscured.
- Treatment—refractory to all treatment:
  - Oral contraceptives for 1–2 years is said to be effective in some cases.

CONCLUSION
Dysmennorhea is a debilitating condition which needs to be paid adequate attention to improve the quality of life for a woman. Reaching a diagnosis of primary or secondary dysmenorrhea and treating the cause goes a long way in ameliorating the condition through expectant, medical and surgical treatment.

SUGGESTED READING
1. Bernardi M, Lazzeri L, Perelli F, et al. Dysmenorrhea and related disorders. 2017; 6:1645.
2. Fauconnier A, Staraci S, Daraï E, et al. A self-administered questionnaire to measure the painful symptoms of endometriosis: Results of a modified DELPHI survey of patients and physicians. J Gynecol Obstet Hum Reprod. 2018;47(2):69-79.
3. Xu Y, Zhao W, Li T, et al. Effects of acupoint—stimulation for the treatment of primary dysmenorrhea compared with NSAIDs: a systematic review and meta-analysis of 19 RCTs. BMC Complement Altern Med. 2017;17(1):436.

CHAPTER 6

Chronic Pelvic Pain

Shweta Mittal Gupta

INTRODUCTION

Chronic pelvic pain (CPP) in women as per Royal College of Obstetricians and Gynecologists (RCOG) is defined as intermittent or constant pain in the lower abdomen or pelvis in a woman of at least 6 months in duration, not occurring exclusively with menstruation or intercourse and not associated with pregnancy. Prevalence of CPP in women aged between 20 and 49 is 15%. Etiology remains unknown in 35–60% of patients. Usually history and pelvic examination are useful in clinching diagnosis. CPP can largely affect social quality of life for the women. Ultrasound forms an important diagnostic modality and endometriosis is one diagnosis which should be kept in mind when dealing with severe chronic pelvic pain. In certain cases laparoscopy helps in not only diagnosis, but also treating endometriosis. Prevalence of chronic pelvic pain ranges from 6% to 27% worldwide. Initial treatment of CPP is usually initiated by gynecologist however it may need a multifactorial and multidisciplinary approach.

Pain is a sensory and emotional experience, which will be affected by physical, social and psychological factors.

HISTORY

It is important for clinician to ask about relationship of pelvic pain with menstrual cycle, aggravating as well as relieving factors. Any relationship of pelvic pain with coitus during micturition or defecation. Thus it becomes important to distinguish if pain is genital, urological, gastrointestinal; musculoskeletal or psychoneurological in origin. Any cyclical pain is usually gynecologic in origin. Pain mapping may be helpful. Patient should localize the pain on a visual representation of the body. This may identify other areas where the patient experiences pain or may reveal a dermatomal distribution, suggesting a nonvisceral source. Chronic pelvic pain can affect social quality of patient's life. Amount of medication patient has been taking to relieve pain should be noted (Table 6.1).

Chronic Pelvic Pain

Table 6.1: History and causes of pelvic pain.

History	Possible causes
Pelvic pain fluctuation with menstrual cycle	Endometriosis or adenomyosis
Crampy pelvic pain	Inflammatory bowel disease, irritable bowel syndrome
Pain during micturition	Interstitial cystitis
Postcoital bleeding	Cervical cancer
Postmenopausal bleed	Endometrial cancer
Prior abdominal surgery	Abdominal adhesion
Unexplained weight loss	Malignancy
Postmenopausal bleed or pain	Malignancy (endometrial)

CAUSES OF CHRONIC PELVIC PAIN

- Deep endometriosis
- Adhesions
- Ovarian cysts
- *Tubal*: Hydrosalpinx, hematosalpinx
- Uterine adenomyosis, fibroids
- Pelvic congestion
- Chronic pelvic inflammatory disease
- *Intestinal pathology*: Colon, appendix, small bowel
- Interstitial cystitis or radiation cystitis
- Nerve entrapment in the wall
- *Malignancies*: Gynecologic, bladder, colon
- Musculoskeletal conditions.

NOTE

- Deep endometriosis is an important cause of pelvic pain and varies markedly over menstrual cycle. Dysmenorrhea, dyspareunia and CPP are the cardinal signs of endometriosis and adenomyosis. Cystic endometriosis causes severe pain in 75% of cases and typical endometriosis causes pain in 50% of cases. Pelvic pain in adenomyosis is variable.
- Acute pain reflects fresh tissue damage and pain disappears after tissue healing. In chronic pelvic pain ever after initial tissue injury the pain may remain for long time which ultimately leads to a modulation in central nervous system magnifying pain.
- Adhesions can cause CPP by organ distension and stretching. Division of dense pelvic adhesions can bring relief in CPP.
- Perihepatic adhesions occurring in pelvic inflammatory disease (PID) can cause pain in liver region during body movement.

- Some hydrosalpinx cause pelvic pain.
- Hydronephrosis can cause pelvic pain originating from renal region.
- Interstitial cystitis is a recognized cause of pelvic pain. Diagnosis is by cystoscopy and confirmed by biopsy.

Make special note of red flag findings (representative of serious systemic disease):
- Postcoital bleed
- Postmenopausal bleed
- Unexplained weight loss
- Adnexal mass
- Gross or microscopic hematuria
- Mass on ultrasound.

PHYSICAL EXAMINATION (TABLE 6.2)

According to the International Pelvic Pain Society detailed history and physical examination needs to be performed along with mapping and quantification of pelvic pain. During physical examination in order to determine origin of pelvic pain a meticulous search for the organ involved or tissue or muscle or dermatome is noted.

To begin with during abdominal examination look for tender points along with surgical scar sites. Notice any vaginal discharge or any vulvar inflammation or growth. Gentle speculum insertion should be performed so that patient does not experience instrumentation pain. Single digit examination using flat end of finger is preferred method and note is made of focal tenderness points, uterine enlargement, uterine movement tenderness and adnexal masses with adnexal tenderness. Physical examination for chronic pelvic is not complete unless tenderness is checked over pubic symphysis or sacroiliac joints and lower back.

Different locations of pain with possible causes (Figs. 6.1 to 6.3).

Table 6.2: Physical examination.	
Physical examination findings	Possible cause
Uterine movement tenderness or enlarged uterus	Adenomyosis, endometritis
Adnexal mass	Ovarian cyst or malignancy
Restricted uterine movement	Endometriosis or adenomyosis
Positive Carnett's sign	Myofascial source of pain
Uterovesical nodularity	Endometriosis
Forniceal tenderness	Pelvic inflammatory disease
Pelvic floor muscle tenderness	Interstitial cystitis

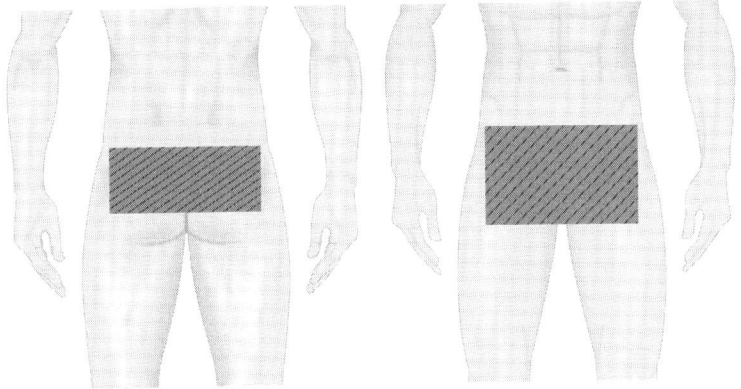

Fig. 6.1: Infraumbilical pain radiating to back.

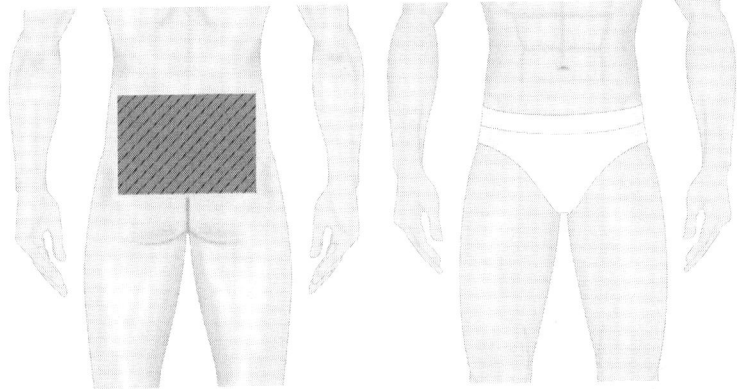

Fig. 6.2: Isolated back pain usually is not gynecological.

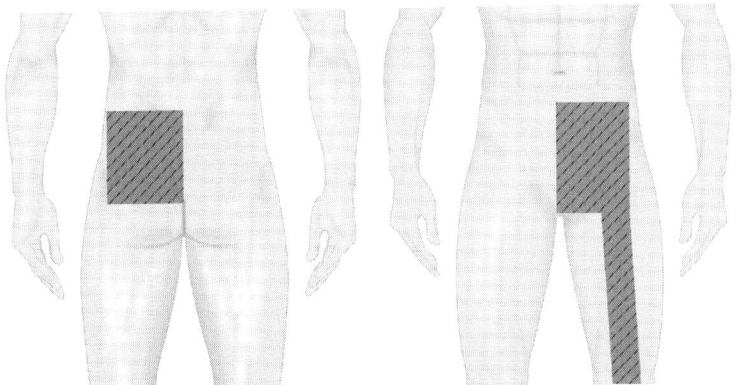

Fig. 6.3: Ovarian cyst can cause pain radiating towards knee and anterior tibial region.

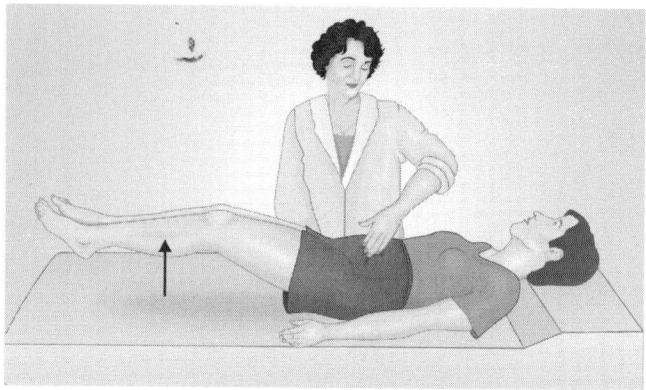

Fig. 6.4: Carnett's test.

Carnett's test is used to differentiate between visceral or myofascial pain (Fig. 6.4). The patient is asked to raise her both legs, while examiner places a finger on painful abdominal site. If the pain increases during this maneuver when rectus abdominis muscles are contracted, it indicates myofascial pain (entrapped nerves or hernia or myositis or trigger points).

DIAGNOSTIC TEST

After a thorough history taking followed by physical examination comes the limited role of diagnostic tests. Usually laboratory testing holds limited value in diagnosing cause of chronic pelvic pain:

- Exclude pregnancy and pregnancy-related complications.
- Complete blood count (CBC) with erythrocyte sedimentation rate (ESR).
- Test for sexually transmitted infections like chlamydia (endocervical sample) or gonorrhea.
- Urine analysis.
- Pelvic ultrasound to detect ovarian or adnexal masses, adenomyosis, hydrosalpinx suggesting PID. Transvaginal ultrasound if of little value in detecting peritoneal endometriosis. Note should be made of probe tenderness or restricted ovarian mobility.
- Magnetic resonance imaging (MRI) usually confirms diagnosis of ultrasound in case of diagnostic dilemma. It can be of special value in case of rectovaginal disease.
- Laparoscopy definitely holds an important diagnostic as well as therapeutic tool especially for endometriosis or pelvic adhesions causing pain. However in today's scenario it is considered as second line management if other therapeutic measures fail.

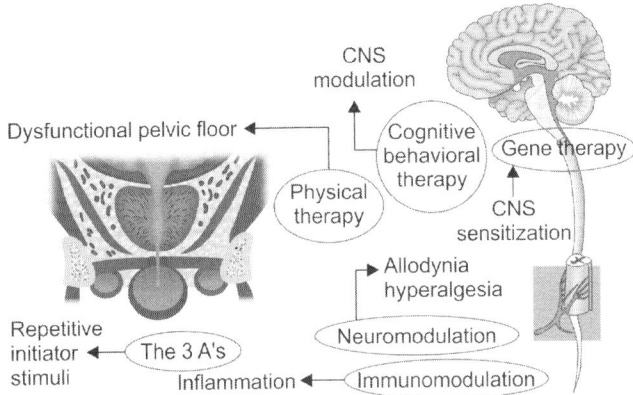

Fig. 6.5: Management of chronic prostatitis or chronic pelvic pain syndrome patient.

MANAGEMENT

Management of chronic pelvic pain remains centered towards making quality of life better for patient and relieving patient symptoms. Since multiple factors could be playing in causing pelvic pains, no specific medication might help. However, a holistic approach encompassing multiple medical management along with need for surgical intervention and if required might be needed. All the aspects such as physical, psychological, sexual and behavioral components need to be addressed (Fig. 6.5).

In the initial management care should be taken of organic, psychological, dietary and environmental causes of pain.

Medical Management

Although nonsteroidal anti-inflammatory are most commonly used, however as per Cochrane review suggested that nonsteroidal anti-inflammatory drug (NSAID) are not effective for chronic pelvic pain.

Pelvic Pain

Women with cyclical pain should be offered hormonal suppression for duration of 3–6 months.

In cases of chronic pelvic pain, progestogens (e.g. medroxyprogesterone depot 150 mg intramuscular (IM) every 3 months could be useful. In suspected endometriosis or adenomyosis different agents found to useful are gonadotropin-releasing hormone (GnRH) depot along with add back therapy to manage side effects of hypoestrogenic situation. Levonorgestrel intrauterine contraceptive device can reduce recurrence of pelvic pain especially after surgery.

Neuropathic Pain

Different drugs used for suspected neuropathic pain are:
- Tricyclic antidepressants (amitriptyline, sertraline, nortriptyline).
- Anticonvulsants (gabapentine, pregabalin, lamotrigine).
- Serotonin-norepinephrine reuptake inhibitors.
- Botulinum toxin.

As per Cochrane review tricyclic antidepressants are effective for chronic pelvic pain and mainstay for managing chronic pelvic pain especially neuropathic pain. Gabapentine used in combination with amitriptyline causes better pain relief than individual drugs. Patients with neurogenic pain respond well to gabapentine and pregabalin also serving as a marker to diagnose neurogenic origin of pain. Antidepressant may alter the pain inhibitory pathway modulating serotonin, noradrenaline, opioidergic or N-methyl-D-aspartate (NMDA) antagonistic effects.

Anticonvulsants act in relieving CPP by inhibition of gamma-aminobutyric acid (GABA) channels and inhibition of voltage gated sodium-potassium channels. Minor side effects such as drowsiness and nausea are frequently seen. While on these medications, they seems to have more beneficial effect in relieving vulvodynia.

Opioids are reserved for nonmalignant pain management only if other drugs fail to improve pain score.

Botulinum toxoid (Botox): Although some studies have shown evidence for using botulinum toxoid injections, however the evidence is still poor. It not only works at local muscular level but also has effect on CNS. In studies it was used for women with more than 2 years of pelvic pain with pelvic floor myalgias.

Melatonin has been used to reduce daily pain, dysuria, dyschezia, menstrual pain. It was found more beneficial in women without endometriosis.

Surgical Management

Laparoscopy

If endometriosis is suspected, then laparoscopic intervention might be needed. Some patients might be benefitted by hysterectomy eventually. This will also help in improving mental, physical health and social functioning. However 40% will still have persistent pain even after hysterectomy.

Before surgery informed consent should detail of the following:
- Superficial endometriosis will be vaporized, ovarian endometriomas will be excised.
- Discuss the extent of adhesiolysis in case of severe adhesions and if adenomyosis is diagnosed (Incomplete excision of deep endometriosis due to lack of experience can cause persistent pelvic pain).

- *Sacral nerve blocks* or neuromodulation have been tried for sacral nerve pains. Laparoscopic uterosacral nerve ablation (LUNA) was frequently used to treat CPP. However, meta-analysis published in 2009 and 2010 concluded that LUNA did not help in alleviating CPP. On the other hand presacral neurectomy involving transection of presacral nerve may be effective for endometriosis induced dysmenorrhea. Care has to be exercised while performing presacral neurectomy to prevent lymphatic and vascular complications; Instead injection of phenol has been tried over presacral neurectomy to destroy presacral nerves.
- *Neuromodulation.*
- Posterior tibial nerve stimulation (PNTS).
- Sacral nerve or root stimulation (SNM).
- Pudendal nerve stimulation.

Posterior tibial nerve stimulation has been used in patients with CPP associated with urge incontinence, urgency or frequency. This can be adopted if other treatment modalities have failed to elicit benefit.

Sacral nerve modulation: It involves implantation of stimulatory device to be implanted at sacral nerve or root. It can have significant complication rate requiring removal of implant and resurgery. This therapy focuses on stimulation of nerve which will act as main driving force for eliciting positive response.

Spinal cord stimulation has been used to treat chronic neuropathic pain in patients resistant to other treatments. Not very useful for sacral nerves and pudendal nerves.

Biofeedback have been used and proposed by some studies to be better than electrostimulation of pelvic floor muscles. Pelvic floor therapies can be considered when treating chronic pelvic pain.

Behavioral therapy will also form an important component while treating chronic pelvic pain. Cognitive psychotherapy and physiotherapy help patient being more aware of their own body image and coping methods as well relieving muscular pains.

Comorbid depression should be dealt alongside chronic pelvic pain. Patients fare better if they receive antidepressants after laparoscopic surgery.

The key role in managing chronic pelvic pain is to understand that CNS plays an important role. Initial treatments should target medical management initially with combinations of drugs if required. Deep endometriosis can be a major gynecological cause of CPP and needs to be dealt. Initial management with anticonvulsants or antidepressants can be started by gynecologist. Further invasive therapies will need specialized pain management team. It is however important for gynecologist to be aware of different approach to manage chronic pelvic pain.

Management of chronic pelvic pain is discussed in Flowchart 6.1.

Flowchart 6.1: Algorithm to manage chronic pelvic pain.

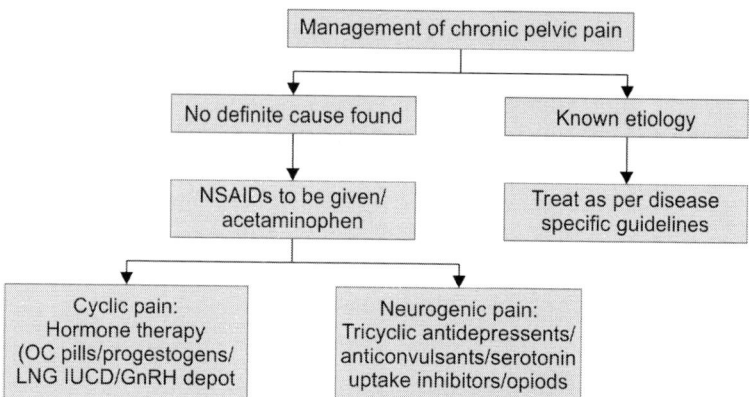

(NSAIDs: nonsteroidal anti-inflammatory drugs; OC: oral contraceptive; LNG: levonorgestrel; IUCD: intrauterine contraceptive device; GnRH: gonadotropin-releasing hormone).

CONCLUSION

Chronic pelvic pain needs multidisciplinary approach and usually is a diagnosis by exclusions. Careful history and meticulous examination can help in diagnosing cause of CPP. Limited investigations are needed and should be performed as and when required. First approach to treat CPP should be medical. Endometriosis forms a major cause of persistent cyclical CPP and even may need surgical intervention to diagnose and treat.

SUGGESTED READING

1. Ortiz DD. Chronic pelvic pain in women. Am Fam Physician. 2008;77(11):1535-42.
2. Speer LM, Mushkbar S, Erbele T. Chronic pelvic pain in women. 2016;93(5):380-7.
3. Royal College of Obstetricians and Gynaecologists. (2012). The initial management of chronic pelvic pain, RCOG, Green top guidelines No.41. [Online] Available from https://www.rcog.org.uk/en/guidelines-research-services/guidelines/gtg41/ [Accessed October, 2018].
4. Royal College of Obstetricians and Gynaecologists. (2015). Therapies targeting the nervous system for chronic pelvic pain, RCOG, Scientific impact paper no.46. [Online] Available from https://www.rcog.org.uk/globalassets/documents/guidelines/scientific-impact-papers/sip46.pdf/ [Accessed October, 2018].

CHAPTER 7

Urinary Problems in Women: Hush No More

Geeta Mediratta

INTRODUCTION

Urinary problems in women are seen from childhood to postmenopausal age group. They are usually temporary and can be managed at outpatient department (OPD). A detailed history and examination is usually sufficient to diagnose the condition. However, specific investigations need to be done in some patients to arrive at an exact diagnosis. The following chapter discusses some common urinary symptoms in women, their diagnosis and management.

Urinary symptoms in women range from leakage of urine to painful urination or blood in urine to painful bladder syndrome to voiding dysfunction. Involuntary leakage of urine in women is a very embarrassing symptom and most women prefer to suffer in silence. In this section the following will be discussed:
- Urinary incontinence
- Voiding dysfunction
- Bladder pain syndrome.

URINARY INCONTINENCE

These refer to involuntary leakage of urine. The impact of leakage of urine can be tremendous in terms of money spent on pads or diapers or surgery. It affects the social life of the women from a minor degree to a major degree, i.e. the "bother index" may vary from very low to high. In case the bother index is high, evaluation and management should be offered. In most women, incontinence can be relieved greatly by using simple exercises or drugs.

TYPES OF DISORDERS

Stress Urinary Incontinence

This refers to leakage of urine during episodes of rise in intra-abdominal pressure, e.g. sneezing, coughing, jumping or exercise. In these situations bladder pressure rises higher than the pressure in the urethra and leakage occurs, i.e. the closure mechanism in the urethra cannot withstand the raised bladder pressure.

Urge Urinary Incontinence and Overactive Bladder

Urge urinary incontinence refers to leakage of the urine which is associated with or preceded by urgency, i.e. strong desire to pass urine. Women also have other complains such as urgency, nocturia, and increased daytime frequency. Nocturia refers to waking up one or more times a night to void. Urgency is the sudden desire to pass urine that is difficult to delay. Detrusor over activity can be of two types.

Neurogenic detrusor over activity: In this case a neurological condition may account for the finding and second is idiopathic detrusor over activity when there is no defined cause.

The term overactive bladder syndromes refer to symptoms of urgency, frequency and urge incontinence. It is referred to as frequency and urgency without urgency incontinence *(OAB-dry)* when there is no leakage of urine and frequency and urgency accompanied by urge incontinence *(OAB-wet)* when there is incontinence of urine.

Mixed Incontinence

This refers to women with symptom of both stress and urge to incontinence and in older women, urge incontinence predominates, while stress incontinence predominates in younger women.

Functional and Transient Incontinence

Functional incontinence is more common in elderly women and refers to leakage due to other factors (nonphysiological). A useful mnemonic to help remember these factors is DIAPPERS.
- **D**: Delirium
- **I**: Infection
- **A**: Atrophic urethritis and vaginitis
- **P**: Pharmacological causes
- **P**: Psychological causes
- **E**: Excessive urine production
- **R**: Restricted mobility
- **S**: Stool impaction.

Extraurethral Incontinence

A traumatic opening between the urinary tract and other genital track is called a fistula. Vesicovaginal fistulas are most common but fistulas may also occur between the vagina, uterus or bowel and the urethra, ureter or bladder.

Vesicovaginal fistulas usually result from obstructed labor. The most common cause of genitourinary fistulas is surgical trauma, malignancy and radiation therapy alone or in combination.

RISK FACTORS FOR URINARY INCONTINENCE

Advanced age, pregnancy, childbirth and obesity, are associated with increased rates of incontinence.

APPROACH TO PATIENT WITH INCONTINENCE

History

The general medical history is important to rule out diabetes mellitus, vascular insufficiency, chronic pulmonary disease and a wide variety of neurologic conditions.

Quality of Life Measures

[Urogenital Distress Inventory (UDI-6), King's Health Questionnaire (KHQ), Incontinence Quality of Life (I-QOL), etc.] can be used to evaluate the impact of incontinence on their lives.

Physical Examination

Neurologic

- Mental status
- Perineal sensation
- Perineal reflexes
- Patellar reflexes.

Abdominal Examination

Masses or fibroids or ovarian cyst.

Cardiovascular Examination

- Congestive heart failure
- Lower extremity edema.

Mobility

Gait assessment.

Pelvic Examination

- Prolapse
- Atrophy

- Levator muscle palpation
- Anal sphincter function.

Test of Urethral Mobility—Q-tip Test

Q-tip test is for determining the degree of urethral mobility with increase in intra-abdominal pressure and more than 45° excursion indicates a hypermobile urethra.

Voiding Diary

A frequency or volume bladder chart is an important aid in the evaluation of patients with urinary incontinence. This chart provides vital information about bladder function, i.e. 24-hour urinary output, the total number of voids, number of nighttime voids, the average voided volume, and the functional bladder capacity.

Urine Analysis

Examination of the urine by dipstick testing and microscopy is done to check for infection, hematuria and metabolic abnormalities. Confirmation by microscopic evaluation is mandatory. Hematuria found in the absence of bacteriuria indicates kidney or bladder tumors.

Postvoid Residual Volume

Large postvoidal residual urine volume indicates diminished functional bladder capacity. Incomplete bladder emptying may cause incontinence.

Cough-Stress Test

This test can be positive in cases of genuine stress urinary incontinence (SUI). However, many women may experience urine loss during coughing due to cough induced detrusor overactivity (urge incontinence).

Pad Tests

These tests quantify the volume of urine lost by weighing the pad before and after activity (24–48 hours).

Urodynamics

This is recommended in the following circumstances:
- The diagnosis is uncertain
- Surgery is being considered
- The patient has hematuria.

Uroflowmetry

This is the graphical representation of the voiding pattern of the patient in which the column of urine voided is plotted over time. Flow time, peak flow rate and mean flow rate are recorded. These increase as the voided volume increases (Figs. 7.1 and 7.2).

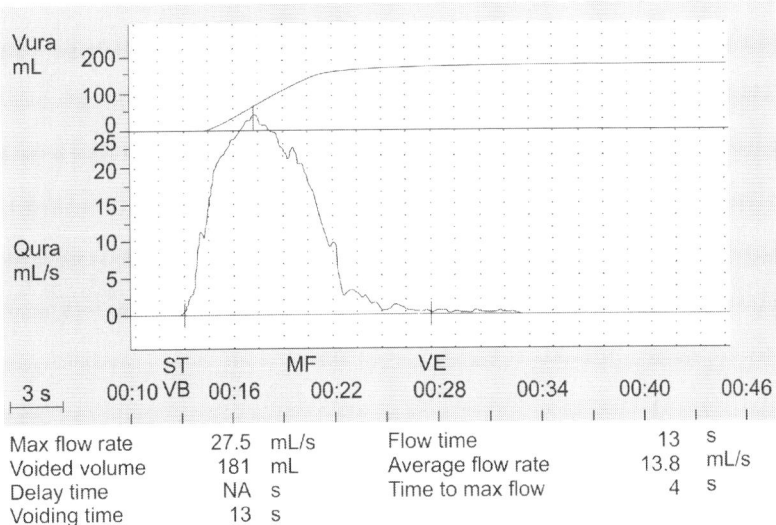

Fig. 7.1: Normal flow.

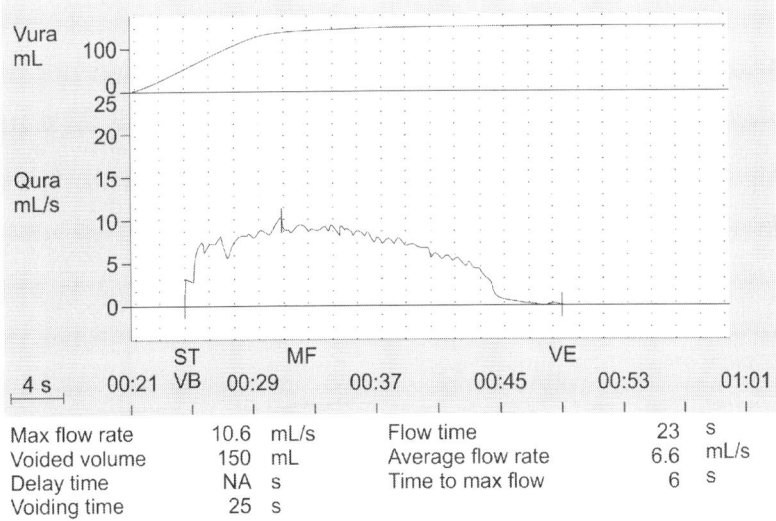

Fig. 7.2: Abnormal flow.

Filling Cystometry

It is done to assess bladder and urethral function during phase of bladder filling and emptying. A close study of the bladder pressures and abdomen pressures in response to filling of the bladder gives valuable information about the physiology. The single channel cystometry is performed. The first sensation occurs at about 100–150 mL of urine followed by bladder capacity of about 400–500 mL of urine. Patients have a strong desire to pass urine at about 600–700 mL of urine depending on the age of the patient. The graph also indicates any uninhibited detrusor contractions leading to feeling of urgency or urge incontinence.

Imaging Tests

Functional magnetic resonance imaging (MRI) is the test of choice for detecting urethral diverticulum.

Neurophysiologic Tests

The neuromuscular function of the pelvic floor is dependent on the integrity of the nervous system.

Pudendal Nerve Terminal Motor Latency

The pudendal nerve terminal motor latency (PNTML) indirectly assesses the integrity and patency of the terminal portion of the pudendal nerve, its neuromuscular junction, and the muscle it serves.

Electromyography

Electromyography (EMG) assesses the inherent electrical potentials generated during neuronal activation of skeletal muscle. This is done by using surface electrodes or needle electrodes and measures the muscle activity in the area of the applied electrode. Currently the main value of the needle EMG is its ability to assess nerve injury and whether the injury is acute or chronic.

NONSURGICAL TREATMENT

Treatment of urinary incontinence can be either nonsurgical or surgical. The approach to treatment is based on the clinical findings and the degree of discomfort experienced by the patient, who should be fully informed of the risks and expected outcome.

Lifestyle Changes

Weight loss in obese women is an important intervention. Postural changes such as crossing the legs during periods of increased abdominal pressure can sometimes prevent increased urinary incontinence. Decreased caffeine intake and decreased fluid intake also helps to some extent.

Physical Therapy

The Cochrane Incontinence Group concluded that pelvic floor muscle training helps to alleviate SUI and should be offered as first line conservative management to women.

The women must be taught to do the Kegel exercise correctly and regularly for an adequate duration, i.e. 3-4 times per week with three repetitions of 8-10 contractions each time.

Behavioral Therapy and Bladder Training

Bladder training focuses on altering bladder function by changing voiding habits and it helps in improving voluntary control rather than bladder function. The main aim of bladder training is a scheduled voiding program. After reviewing the patient's voiding diary, an initial voiding interval is chosen that is equal to the longest interval between voiding that is comfortable.

The patient is then told to empty her bladder when she awakes and then everytime during the day when that interval is reached. In case the women feels like voiding during that interval, she is instructed to use urge suppression technique such as clenching and unclenching the hands, wiggling the toes, doing a mental mathematics or doing deep breathing. Another method is to contract the pelvic floor muscles several times in a row. This training should continue for 6 weeks before results are seen.

The primary technique of behavioral training is pelvic floor muscle training, but with a focus on urge inhibition.

Patients with neurogenic detrusor overactivity and do not respond as well to behavioral therapy because the problem is related to neural pathway destruction.

Vaginal Devices

Vaginal devices (pessaries) and urethral inserts are available for treating SUI, e.g. incontinence ring with support, incontinence dish, etc. There are not of proven benefit in all patients, only some women benefit.

Medications

Stress Incontinence

The tone of the urethra and bladder neck is maintained in large part by α-adrenergic activity from the sympathetic nervous system. Currently, serotonin norepinephrine reuptake inhibitors (SNRIs) are being used. Duloxetine chloride 40 mg/day is commonly being used with a 59-60% reduction in incontinence episode frequency.

Urge Incontinence and Overactive Bladder

These drugs are anticholinergic agents that exert their effects on the bladder by blocking the activity of acetylcholine at muscarinic receptor sites. Commonly used medications are:

- Oxybutynin 2.5-5 mg TID—QID
- Tolteridine 1-2 mg BD (immediate release) and 4 mg once (extended release)
- Solifenacin succinate 5-20 mg once a day
- Mirabegron 25-50 mg once daily.

In general, the drug reduces incontinence episodes by 50-70%, whereas placebo reduces incontinence episodes by 40-60%.

When initiating therapy it is best to start with a lower dose (particularly for elderly patients) and increase it as needed to a higher, more frequent dose (2.5-5 mg) TDS—QID.

Patients must be informed about the side effects of anticholinergic agents like dry mouth and constipation. They must be told that this is not due to thirst. Some patients increase their fluid intake to combat this problem with a subsequent worsening of their incontinence. The patient can be told to treat dry mouth by chewing gum or eating a piece of moist fruit rather than drinking water. Elderly women should be carefully evaluated for open angle glaucoma before giving these drugs.

Mirabegron 25-50 mg once a day is a new drug for overactive bladder. This acts as a β-3 adrenergic receptor agonist and has a very good safety profile in elderly patients.

Nocturia and Nocturnal Enuresis

This is very common in children and elderly. Medications that treat nocturia and nocturnal enuresis cause either:

- To reduce urine output
- To increase in bladder capacity and reduce unstable bladder contractions
- To act centrally on sleep and micturition centers.

Tricyclic antidepressants, particularly imipramine are being used and they work by changing sleep mechanism, by providing anticholinergic or antidepressant effects, or by affecting antidiuretic hormone excretion. The dose of imipramine is 25 mg at bedtime.

SURGICAL TREATMENT FOR STRESS INCONTINENCE

- Retropubic urethropexy (colposuspension)
- Traditional pubovaginal sling
- Minimally invasive sling
- Bulking agents
- Tension free vaginal tape (retropubic and transobturator tape).

Currently the treatment of SUI has revolved around this technique that has now superceded the older method of Burch colposuspension and Marshall-Marchetti-Krantz procedure which had a success rate of 70–80%.

A great deal of well-designed trials have proven the superiority of transobturator tapes which is placed in a tension free manner at the midurethral site to treat stress urinary incontinence (subjective cure rate 80–85% with only 2–3% erosion rate). Rate of bladder perforations is practically nil with this approach. Around 3% incidence of voiding disorders is reported in various trials.

SURGICAL TREATMENT FOR DETRUSOR OVERACTIVITY

Neuromodulation (InterStim)

Women with refractory over active bladder need neuromodulation. Sacral nerve stimulation therapy is performed in two phases. Firstly, upper cutaneous nerve test is performed to determine which patient responds to this type of therapy. Those women who respond are then implanted with permanent electrode lead adjacent to the 3rd sacral nerve root connected to a pulse generator.

Botox Injections

Botulinum toxin A (BTX A), a neurotoxin produced by the anaerobic bacteria *Clostridium botulinum*, acts on peripheral cholinergic nerve endings to inhibit calcium mediated release of acetylcholine vesicles at the presynaptic neuromuscular junction.

This procedure is done via cystoscopy and Botox is injected at 15–30 different detrusor muscle sites under direct visualization, sparing the bladder trigone and the ureteral orifices. This procedure needs to be repeated after 6–8 months and is a promising treatment for overactive bladder.

Augmentation Cystoplasty and Urinary Diversion

These surgical options include:
- Conduit diversion (creation of various intestinal conduits to the skin) or continent diversion (which includes a rectal reservoir or continent cutaneous diversion)
- Bladder reconstruction
- Replacement of the bladder with various intestinal segments
- With the advent of sacral modulation these procedures are done less frequently now.

SURGICAL TREATMENT OF FISTULA

A variety of techniques are available for surgical treatment of fistula, i.e. abdominal repair, vaginal repair and robotic repair.

Cystoscopy

Cystoscopy can be considered in the following circumstances:
- In women with urge incontinence to rule out other disorders, especially in women with microscopic hematuria.
- In the evaluation of vesicovaginal fistula.
- Intraoperatively to evaluate possible ureteral or vesical injury.

VOIDING DYSFUNCTION

Women are affected less commonly compared to men with voiding difficulties. Voiding dysfunction is defines as emptying dysfunction resulting from poor or incomplete relaxation of the pelvic floor muscles or failure of the detrusor muscle to contract appropriately. For normal voiding to occur, the pelvic floor and the urethral sphincter must relax and this should occur along with coordinated contraction of the detrusor muscle that leads to complete bladder emptying. Some women empty their bladders by abdominal straining in the absence of a detrusor contraction or by relaxing the pelvic floor. Some women may empty their bladders completely by this method but this is not considered normal voiding pattern as this takes great effort and long time.

Causes

Neurological diseases, e.g. multiple sclerosis causes detrusor sphincter dyssynergia (DSD), i.e. the urethral sphincter contracts at the same time as the detrusor and thus the patient voids with an interrupted stop and start stream and usually has a significant amount of residual urine.

Other causes of voiding difficulties are—antihistaminics, anticholinergics, herpes simplex virus infection, urinary tract infection, obstruction (following bladder neck surgeries or women with advanced pelvic organ prolapse), over distension, severe constipation and psychogenic factors.

Fowler's syndrome refers to unexplained urinary retention occurring as an isolated phenomenon in women 25–30 years of age. The first retention episode is usually triggered by some event like surgery for child birth.

Evaluation

Careful pelvic examination to rule out prolapse and the pelvic masses especially anterior wall myomas are important.

Detailed neurological examination should be done to rule multiple sclerosis and tabes dorsalis. Anal wink reflex and clitoral reflex must be elicited. Patients gait must be assessed.

Urodynamic evaluation helps to determine whether the women have an obstruction type voiding pattern or there is poor contraction of the detrusor muscle.

Cystourethroscopy may be needed to reveal an obstructive lesion such as polyp, obstructive lesion, tumor, ureterocele or ball valve stone.

Treatment

The main thrust of the treatment of voiding difficulty is clean, intermittent self-catheterization. Self-catheterization allows the patient to do this task using a small (14-Fr) plastic catheter that patient inserts through the urethra into the bladder, draining its contents. The catheter is then removed, washed with soap and water, dried and stored in a clean and dry place.

In addition neuromodulation of the sacral nerve roots may also help women with nonobstructive urine retention.

For patients who are unable to generate a detrusor contraction, bethanechol chloride (cholinergic agonist) has been used in doses of 25 mg/day.

BLADDER PAIN SYNDROMES

These are disorders of bladder sensation where the patients experience pain rather than lack of bladder sensation. These disorders are amongst the most frustrating urogynecological conditions to manage.

Terminology and Prevalence

Interstitial cystitis or painful bladder syndrome is defined as suprapubic pain related to bladder filling accompanied by other symptoms such as increased daytime and nighttime frequency in the absence of proven urinary infection or other obvious pathology. In other words urgency and pain are the defining characteristics of the painful bladder syndrome.

The prevalence of painful bladder syndrome varies widely depending on the diagnostic criteria used. When mild and moderate cases are considered, the syndrome is quite common, average prevalence being 1 in 5 women.

Diagnosis

Careful history, urine analysis, urine culture is important to diagnose this condition. This is a diagnosis of exclusion therefore other possible causes for painful voiding must be ruled out, e.g. urinary tract infection, vulval disease, endometriosis, urethral diverticula, chemical irritation from bubble baths, soaps or feminine hygiene products, urinary stones, urogenital atrophy from estrogen deprivation and sexually transmitted diseases.

Treatment

The management of painful bladder syndrome focuses on treatment of symptoms. This includes urinary tract analgesics, local hygiene and careful voiding regimen similar to that used in the treatment of detrusor overactivity.

Patients may be advised to eliminate alcohol, tomato, spices, chocolates, caffeine and high acid foods as these cause bladder irritation and inflammation. It is also important to instruct the patient to avoid body powders, perfumes or colored irritating soaps and tight fitting undergarments.

Hydrodistention of the bladder under anesthesia along with instillation of heparin and lignocaine, hydrocortisone and normal saline and sodium bicarbonate.

Because it has been theorized that bladder pain may result from increased histamine release, some patients benefit from medications that block these inflammatory mediators, such as diphenhydramine hydrochloride 25–50 mg orally three times per day in combination with cimetidine 300 mg three times per day. Tricyclic antidepressants help some women by modulating sensory nerve pain. Ongoing preliminary research suggests that some women with severe bladder pain syndrome may find relief following sacral neuromodulation (interStim) or acupuncture.

CONCLUSION

- Urinary symptoms in women range from leakage of urine to painful urination or blood in urine to painful bladder syndrome to voiding dysfunction.
- Urinary incontinence is of two types—stress urinary incontinence and urge urinary incontinence.
- Stress incontinence is the most common type of urinary continence in women; however urge incontinence is the most common type of incontinence in older women.
- Initial evaluation includes detailed history, physical examination, quality of life questionnaire; urine analysis and postvoid residual urine analysis.
- Urodynamic tests are also indicated in certain groups of women like those with mixed incontinence and previous failed anticontinence surgery.
- Treatment of urinary incontinence can be either nonsurgical or surgical.
- In nonsurgical treatment, lifestyle changes, physical therapy, behavioral therapy and bladder training are offered.
- Medications are used in case of failure of above and include duloxetine for stress urinary incontinence and anticholinergic drugs for urge incontinence and overactive bladder.
- Surgical treatment for stress urinary incontinence are retropubic urethropexy, traditional pubovaginal slings, minimally invasive slings, bulking agents and tension free vaginal tape (retropubic and transobturator tape).
- Tension free vaginal tape is the most preferred treatment now.
- The next important urinary problem women face is voiding dysfunction and it is mainly due to neurologic disease, pelvic organ prolapsed, UTI and drugs like antihistaminics and anticholinergic.

- Bladder pain disorder syndrome is disorder of bladder sensation where the patient experiences pain rather than lack of bladder sensation. These disorders are amongst the most frustrating urogynecological conditions to manage.
- Treatment consists of identifying the cause and treatment accordingly.

SUGGESTED READING

1. American College of Obstetricians and Gynecologists. ACOG Practice Bulletin No. 63: Urinary Incontinence in Women. Obstet Gynecol. 2005;105:1533-45.
2. Bent AE, Cundiff GW, Swift SE. Ostergard's Urogynecology and Pelvic Floor Dysfunction, 6th edition. Philadelphia: Lippincott Williams and Wilkins; 2007.
3. Haylen BT, de Ridder D, Freeman RM, et al. An International Urogynecological Association (IUGA)/International Continence Society (ICS) Joint Report on the Terminology for Female Pelvic Floor Dysfunction. Int Urogynecol J. 2010;21(1):5-26.
4. National Collaborating Centre for Women's and Children's Health. Urinary Incontinence in Women: The Management of Urinary Incontinence in Women. London: Royal College of Obstetricians and Gynecologists (UK); 2013.

CHAPTER 8

Fibroids: A Close Insight

Kanwal Gujral, Pramod Yerne, Anurag Vashista

INTRODUCTION

- Fibroids or leiomyomas are the most common benign tumors of smooth muscle of uterus.
- Incidence is 12.8/1,000 women years.
- Women in reproductive age group have a lifetime incidence of 70%. In other words, 7-8 out of 10 women will have fibroids in their lifetime. Only 25% are symptomatic. Size can vary from pea size to as large as a full term pregnant uterus.

RISK FACTORS

Increased risk is seen with:
- Younger age group
- Infertility
- Obesity
- Polycystic ovarian syndrome
- Hyperestrogenic status
- Oral contraceptive pills started before the age of 16 years.

Reduced risk is seen with:
- Smoking
- Multiparity.

SIGNS AND SYMPTOMS

- About 75% are asymptomatic.
- Most common presenting symptom is abnormal uterine bleeding in the form of heavy menstrual loss, frequent periods and/or irregular periods. This can result into significant anemia.
- Pressure symptoms in the form of urinary frequency, dysuria and urinary retention are seen in few. Occasionally due to back pressure, hydronephrosis can result.

- Infertility is seen in around 2–3% of cases.
- Pelvic pain, mass and constipation are other symptoms.
- Pregnancy with fibroids have risk of abortion, preterm labor, growth restriction, abnormal presentation, red degeneration, prolonged and obstructed labor, higher incidence of cesarean section and postpartum hemorrhage.

CLASSIFICATION

Depending on site, International Federation of Gynecology and Obstetrics (FIGO) has reported a classification given in Box 8.1 and Figure 8.1.

DIAGNOSIS

Diagnosis is mainly by imaging. The most common modality used is transabdominal and/or transvaginal ultrasound that can determine site,

Box 8.1: International Federation of Gynecology and Obstetrics (FIGO) classification of leiomyomas.

SM: Submucosal
0: Pedunculated intracavitary
1: <50% intramural
2: ≥50% intramural

O: Others
3: Contacts endometrium; 100% intramural
4: Intramural
5: Subserosal ≥50% intramural
6: Subserosal <50% intramural
7: Subserosal pedunculated
8: Others (specify, e.g. cervical, parasitic).

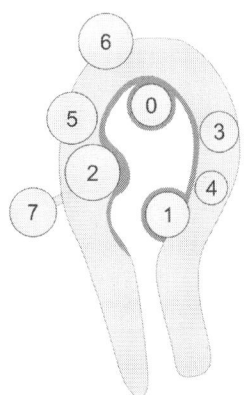

Fig. 8.1: Diagrammatic presentation of International Federation of Gynecology and Obstetrics (FIGO) classification of leiomyomas.

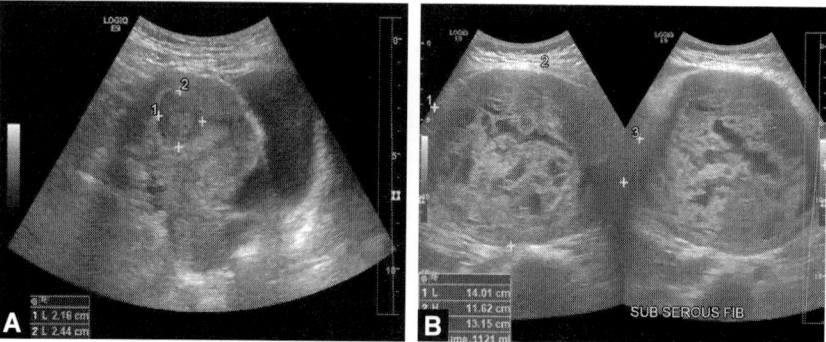

Figs. 8.2A and B: Ultrasound images. (A) Submucosal fibroid; (B) Subserosal fibroid.

number, size and shape of leiomyomas with reasonable accuracy. Ultrasound can also differentiate fibroids from ovarian masses. Saline sonography helps to delineate intracavitary fibroids. Occasionally MRI is needed for mapping of fibroids prior to surgical intervention. It is a good modality to differentiate leiomyomas from adenomyosis (Figs. 8.2A and B).

MANAGEMENT OF FIBROIDS

It depends upon patient's age; desire to preserve fertility, menstrual functions, severity and type of symptoms and size and location of fibroids. Management ranges from simple observation to medical and surgical intervention.

Asymptomatic Fibroids

- Only observation is required.
- Annual checkup with pelvic examination, cervical screening (Pap smear) and ultrasonography (USG) is recommended.
- Neither medical nor surgical intervention is indicated.

Symptomatic Fibroids

Surgical Management

- Surgery is the definitive treatment.
- It involves hysterectomy, i.e. removal of uterus or myomectomy, i.e. removal of fibroids.

Hysterectomy:
- Recommended for symptomatic women in perimenopausal and post-menopausal period.
- Approaches are vaginal, laparoscopic and abdominal depending upon size and expertise of surgeon.

- Vaginal hysterectomy can be accomplished up to 12–14 weeks uterus size.
- Laparoscopic hysterectomy in today's era of minimally invasive surgery is possible in uteri of all sizes, even up to 30 cm by experienced surgeons.
- However, need for morcellation in order to retrieve the uterus must be discussed and consent should be obtained from the patient.
- Morcellation involves fragmenting or breaking the solid uterus into small fragments by electromechanical device. The spillage of morcellated specimen can lead to dissemination in the event of occult malignancy, although reported incidence is only 0.02%.

Myomectomy:
- Procedure of choice for younger women who wish to preserve fertility and also for women who want to preserve their menstrual functions.
- The procedures are:
    - *Hysteroscopic myomectomy:* Ideal procedure for type 0 and type 1 fibroids.
    - *Laparoscopic myomectomy:* For type 2–4 fibroids.
    - Abdominal myomectomy: Preferable for very large fibroids.
- Laparoscopic approach for myomectomy or hysterectomy has advantage of lesser pain, early recovery, shortened hospital stay, early return to work besides cosmetic advantage of a small scar (Figs. 8.3A to C).
- Robotics is the newer addition and is surgeon friendly.

Medical Management

Goal of medical management is:
- To alleviate symptoms, predominantly menstrual loss and improve the quality of life.
- To reduce size and maintain size.
- Have minimal side effects.
- To avoid rebound increase in size.

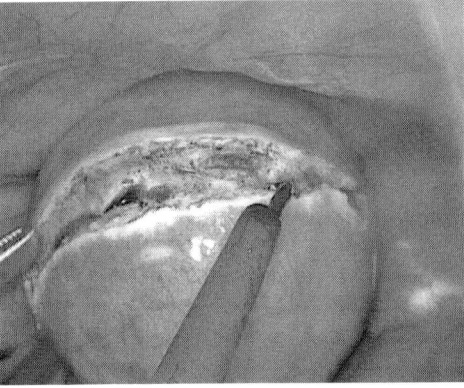

Fig. 8.3A: Laparoscopic myomectomy shows incision on myoma.
(For Color Version, See Color Plate 1)

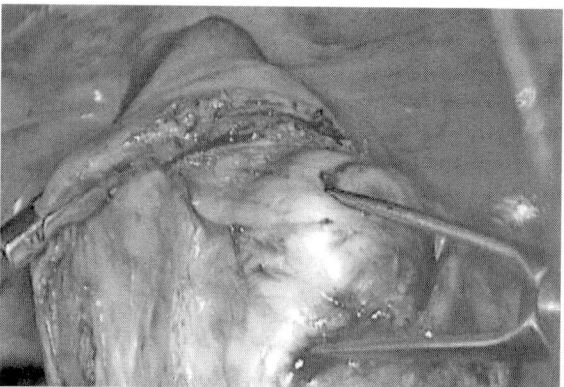

Fig. 8.3B: Laparoscopic myomectomy shows enucleation of myoma.
(For Color Version, See Color Plate 1)

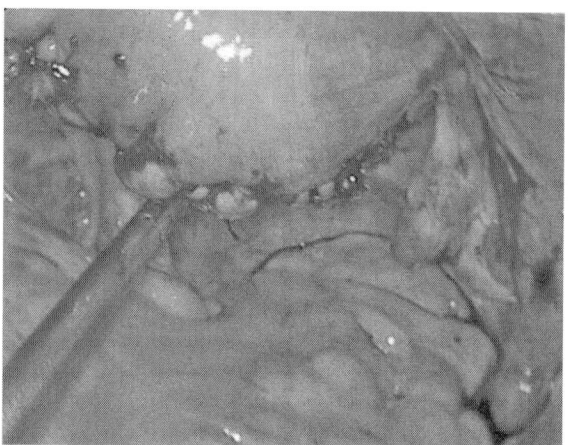

Fig. 8.3C: Laparoscopic myomectomy shows closure of myoma bed.
(For Color Version, See Color Plate 1)

Indications of medical management:
- *Preoperative use*: To reduce menstrual loss and improve hemoglobin.
- To decrease size so as to facilitate laparoscopic approach for surgery or convert abdominal approach to laparoscopic or vaginal approach.
- Decreased size facilitates hysteroscopic myomectomy because of reduced blood flow. However, tissue planes may not be smooth.
- As a temporary measure in women approaching menopause who want to defer surgery.
  Medical treatment can be hormonal or nonhormonal.

Table 8.1: Food and Drug Administration (FDA) approved drugs.

Trade name	Generic name	Dosage	Route	Timing
Lupride	Leuprolide acetate	3.75 mg 11.25 mg	IM or SC IM or SC	Monthly 3 monthly
Decapeptyl	Triptorelin	3.7 mg	IM	Monthly
Zoladex	Goserelin	3.6 mg	IM	Monthly
Zoladex implant	Goserelin	10.6 mg	Implant	–

(IM: intramuscularly; SC: subcutaneously)

Hormonal: Preoperative use.

Gonadotropin-releasing hormone (GnRh) agonists:
- Only Food and Drug Administration (FDA) approved drug for pre-operative reduction in size and symptoms (Table 8.1).
- Fibroid volume is reduced by 30–50% in first 3 months of use.
- Symptoms relief is in 80%.
- Recommended use for 6 months if fibroids are more than 10 cm.
- Side effects:
  - They are related to estrogen deficiency—hot flushes, insomnia, mood changes, vaginal dryness, decreased libido and most importantly, a decrease in bone mineral density (5% at 6 months of use). Initial flare of signs and symptoms may occur.
  - To prevent bone loss, add back therapy in the form of cyclic estrogen and progesterone or combined pills or daily tibolone 2.5 mg is recommended.

Gonadotropin-releasing hormone antagonists:
- No significant advantage over agonists in reducing size or symptoms.
- Cost is exuberant. Daily dosing is another drawback.

To alleviate symptoms and signs:
- *Selective progesterone receptor modulators (SPRMs)*:
  - Ulipristal acetate (UPA): Newer drug showing promising results. It has undergone three phase trial (PEARL trial).

Phase I trial:
- Ulipristal acetate compared to placebo.
- Significant reduction in size and blood loss with UPA.

Phase II trial:
- Ulipristal acetate 5–10 mg compared to leuprolide (3 monthly).
- Ulipristal acetate resulted in amenorrhea earlier by 2 weeks and significant reduction in size and bleeding as compared to leuprolide.

Phase III trial:
- Ulipristal acetate (10 mg) intermittent 12 weeks use for 18 months separated by spontaneous withdrawal or with nor ethisterone.

- About 80% of women experienced amenorrhea and 72% a reduction in volume.

Phase IV trial:

Is evaluating 5 mg or 10 mg for 12 weeks separated by 2 menstrual cycles.

Trade name: Fibroprist, Fibristal.

- *Dosage*:
  - 5 mg once daily for 12 weeks with gap of 2 menstrual cycles.
  - Can be used up to 18 months.
  - For preoperative reduction, short-term use of 3 months.
  - Can be used instead of leuprolide.
- *Advantages*:
  - Minimal hypoestrogenic effects because it maintains estradiol (E2) levels of 50 pg/dL required to maintain bone mineral density.
  - No initial flare up unlike leuprolide.
- *Side effects*:
  - Headache, breast tenderness.
  - Physiological endometrial hyperplasia which is detected on ultrasound as increased endometrial thickness. This does not increase risk of malignancy.
  - Four cases of severe liver injury leading to liver transplantation have been reported, though baseline liver function status was not known in these cases. Therefore, it is advisable to test for serum transaminase levels before starting Ulipristal. Serum transaminases should be tested monthly and drug should be discontinued if the levels reach two-times the upper limit of normal. However, Central Drug Standard Control Organization of India has approved its use in March 2018.

Mifepristone:
- Antiprogesterone drug.
- Less effective than UPA.
- Dose: 5–25 mg daily for 12 weeks.
- Higher relief with higher dose.
- Higher efficacy at dose 50 mg.
- *Side effects*:
  - Hot flushes (38%), endometrial hyperplasia (25%) with use over 6 months.

Levonorgestrel (LNG-IUS):
- Intrauterine device containing 38 mg of LNG releasing 20 µg of LNG per day. Recommended use is for 3–5 years.
- *Indications*:
  - Effective for women who have heavy menstrual loss with fibroid not distorting cavity.

- ♦ Relieves dysmenorrhea.
- ♦ Women who desire contraception along with.
- ♦ Women who prefer one-time method and are not willing to take daily medications.
- *Disadvantages*:
  - ♦ Does not reduce size
  - ♦ Expulsion rate 12%.

Combined oral contraceptive pills:
- Cyclic use from day 5 to day 25 of cycle.
- Effective for short time use in women with heavy menstrual loss due to fibroids.
- No effect on size or other associated symptoms.
- *Dose*: From day 5 of cycle to day 25 of cycle.

Danazol and gestrinone:
- Both are effective for short-term use 4–6 months in reducing menstrual blood loss and dysmenorrhea.
- Less effective in size reduction than GnRH agonist.
- *Dosage*: Danazole: 100–400 mg/day.

Gestrinone: 2.5 mg twice a week for 6 months.
- *Side effects*: Weight gain, headache, muscle cramps, androgenicity, acne, hirsutism, voice change, etc. Hence not preferred.

Other drugs:
- Letrozole (aromatase inhibitor), cabergoline—need larger data to recommend the use.

Nonhormonal:
- *Tranexamic acid*: 2–4 g/day for 4–7 days of cycle reduces menstrual loss by 30–50%. No significant side effects.
- *Nonsteroidal anti-inflammatory drugs (NSAIDs)*: Mefenamic acid: similar effectiveness and better at controlling dysmenorrhea.
- *Vitamin D*: Some recent studies have observed that women with adequate level of vitamin D have 32% lower risk of developing uterine fibroids:
  - ♦ Vitamin D levels have an inverse relation with fibroid volume. Further research is needed to evaluate its efficacy in treating fibroid.

However, vitamin D supplementation may be used as a preventive approach in vitamin D deficient individuals.

Interventional Radiology

Uterine artery embolization (UAE):
- It is a procedure which occludes the vascular supply to fibroids resulting in infarction and absorption.

Flowchart 8.1: Management of types of fibroids.

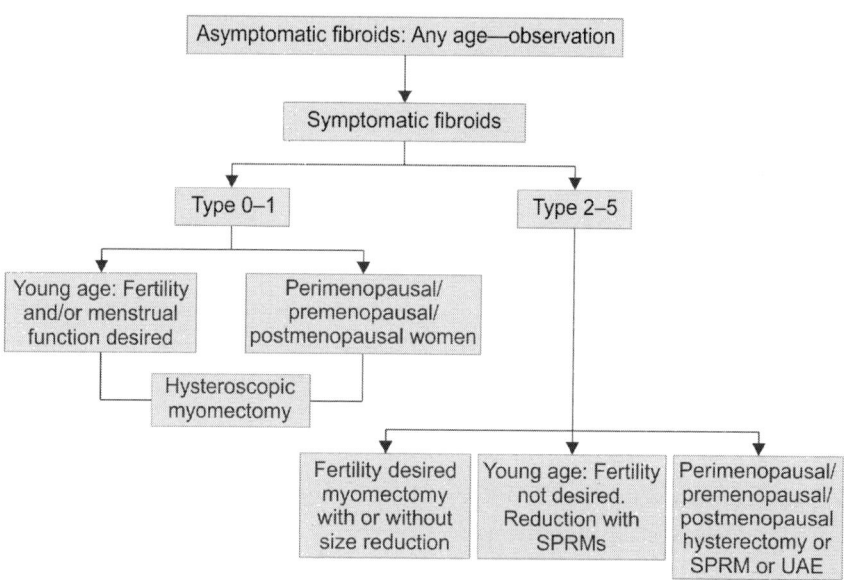

(SPRMs: selective progesterone receptor modulators; UAE: uterine artery embolization)

- It should be considered in women with symptomatic fibroids who do not desire pregnancy.
- Fibroids of any size and location can be treated by UAE.
- Procedure is done under local anesthesia by cannulating femoral artery and reaching up to uterine artery under fluoroscopic guidance and injecting embolics.
- Procedure takes 1–1.5 hours.
- Side effects in the form of pain, limb edema, etc. are of minor variety.
- If women desire fertility, UAE is not a choice over myomectomy as it causes decreased ovarian reserve.

High Frequency Magnetic Resonance-guided Focused Ultrasound Energy (MRgFUS)

- It is a method by which ultrasound energy is directed to a point inside the myoma and coagulative tissue necrosis is induced. It is a new method, safety data is scarce and additional work is needed to recommend its routine use.
- Management summary is depicted in the Flowchart 8.1.

CONCLUSION

- Uterine fibroids or leiomyomas are the most common benign tumors of smooth muscle of the uterus.

- Myoma size can vary from a pea size to as large as a full-term pregnant uterus.
- Only about one-third of women are symptomatic. Common symptoms are abnormal uterine bleeding, urinary symptoms, backache, pelvic pressure and pain. Infertility is seen in 2–3% of cases.
- Management depends upon patients' age, desire to preserve fertility or menstrual function, severity of symptoms, size and location of fibroids.
- Asymptomatic fibroids only need to be observed with annual checkup.
- For symptomatic fibroids, medical and surgical management are the options.
- Conservative surgical management is myomectomy—hysteroscopic, laparoscopic or by laparotomy.
- Definite surgical management is by hysterectomy.
- Medical management is an alternative to surgical management for women who do not desire fertility, are young and want to preserve their menstrual function. Out of the armamentarium of medical therapy, SPRMs have the best results with least side effects.
- Uterine artery embolization is another alternative to surgery in selected few.

SUGGESTED READING

1. Contributors: Modern management of fibroids. Clinical Obstetrics and Gynecology. South Holland: Wolters Kluwer; 2016.
2. Donnez J, Dolmans MM. Uterine fibroid management: from the present to the future. Hum Reprod Update. 2016;22(6):665-86.
3. Marret H, Fritel X, Ouldamer L, et al. Therapeutic management of uterine fibroid tumors: updated French guidelines. Eur J Obstet Gynecol Reprod Biol. 2012;165(2):156-64.
4. Pérez-López FR, Ornat L, Ceausu I, et al. EMAS position statement: management of uterine fibroids. Maturitas. 2014;79(1):106-16.
5. Uterine fibroids from pathogenesis to clinical management. Best Practice and Research Clinical Obstetrics and Gynecology. Amsterdam: Elsevier Ltd; 2016.

CHAPTER 9

When to Intervene in a Case of Ovarian Cyst?

Kanika Jain, Kanika Chopra

INTRODUCTION

Ovarian cysts occur commonly in woman of all ages. Majority are asymptomatic, few presenting with pain or pelvic symptoms. Ovarian cyst inevitably raises the question of its relevance to women's symptoms and concern for the possibility of ovarian malignancy, both in the minds of the patient and her treating physician. But, definitely not all ovarian cysts, whether in premenopausal or postmenopausal women require surgical intervention. So, it is the need of hour to have appropriate knowledge of the subject. The diagnosis of the cause of ovarian cyst in a woman varies with the age of presentation, although overlap of differential diagnosis does exist (Tables 9.1 and 9.2).

FUNCTIONAL OVARIAN CYSTS

- Functional cysts are of two types—follicular cyst and corpus luteal cyst.
- These cysts have complex pathogenesis and are usually due to alteration in the release of anterior pituitary hormones, more commonly known as hormonal imbalance.

Table 9.1: Types of ovarian mass.

Benign ovarian cysts	<ul><li>Functional cysts</li><li>Endometriomas</li><li>Serous cystadenomas</li><li>Mucinous cystadenomas</li><li>Mature teratomas</li><li>Paraovarian cysts</li><li>Tubo-ovarian complexes</li></ul>
Primary malignant ovarian	<ul><li>Germ cell tumors</li><li>Epithelial cell carcinoma</li><li>Sex-cord stromal tumors</li></ul>
Secondary malignant ovarian	<ul><li>Predominantly breast, endometrial and gastrointestinal carcinomas</li></ul>

When to Intervene in a Case of Ovarian Cyst?

Table 9.2: Histological classification of all ovarian neoplasm.

Coelomic epithelium	- Serous - Mucinous - Endometrioid - Brenner
Gonadal stroma	- Granulosa theca - Sertoli-Leydig - Lipid cell fibroma
Germ cell	- Dysgerminoma - Teratoma - Endodermal sinus (yolk sac) - Choriocarcinoma
Miscellaneous	- Lymphoma - Sarcoma
Metastatic	- Colorectal - Breast - Endometrial

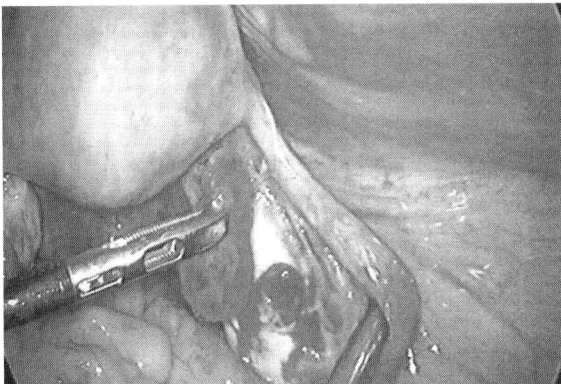

Fig. 9.1: Functional cyst seen in ovary. *(For Color Version, See Color Plate 2)*

- Usually patients present with mild-to-moderate unilateral pain lower abdomen and alternation in menstrual cycle. These can be managed conservatively in majority of the cases.
- The third least common is the theca lutein cysts, which are usually seen in association with twin pregnancy, gestational trophoblastic disease, or in association with ovulation induction with clomiphene citrate and gonadotropins. They usually resolve on their own (Fig. 9.1).

BENIGN OVARIAN NEOPLASM

- About 25% of ovarian cysts in reproductive age group are nonfunctional ovarian neoplasm.

- Most common of these are serous cystadenomas. Among these, 70% are benign, 10% have low malignant potential, and rest 20% are frankly malignant. In these cases, usually oophorectomy is done.
- The second in this list is mucinous cystadenomas, and around 15% of these turn malignant.
- Endometrioid tumors form the third most common type and take the form of endometriomas. Endometriomas can be primary or secondary. Primary endometriomas originate by the invagination of surface endometrial glands and secondary originate in functional cysts. These are usually symptomatic and require surgical intervention.
- The solid ovarian tumor in this list is the Brenner tumor, and is more commonly seen in older woman in association with mucinous cystadenomas.
- Among germ cell tumors, dermoid cyst is the most common and is usually seen around 30 years of age. They usually have acute presentation due to increased risk of torsion owing to the increased fat content of these masses. Dermoid cysts are seen in 70% of cases in reproductive age group, and developed from single primordial germ cells. It comprises of all three germ cells—ectoderm, endoderm, and mesoderm. This requires surgical management (Fig. 9.2).
- Stromal cell tumors are a group of solid tumors and constitute granulose theca cell tumors and Sertoli-Leydig cell tumors. These are functional tumors producing hormones and resulting in symptoms accordingly.
- Ovarian fibroma is another subset of tumors, which are solid tumors, of sex cord stromal tumor variety and is seen to be associated with ascites and pleural effusion in some patients, more commonly known as Meig's syndrome. Surgical management is required in all these cases.

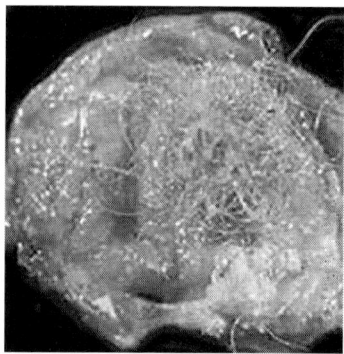

Fig. 9.2: Cut section image of a dermoid cyst. *(For Color Version, See Color Plate 2)*

MALIGNANT OVARIAN NEOPLASM

- Ovarian malignancy is the most common cause of death from gynecological cancers in women, due to its late detection. About two-thirds of patients have advanced disease at the time of presentation.
- Usually, it is seen in 5th to 6th decade of life.
- The common predisposing factors are nulliparity, primary infertility, endometriosis, and family history.
- These can be of epithelial, germ cell, sex cord, mixed, or secondary from a primary lesion elsewhere in the body.
- Majority of the ovarian malignancies are of epithelial cell type, which is around 90%. Serous cystadenocarcinomas are the most common type.
- Mucinous cystadenocarcinomas are the second most common type and are known to assume huge sizes.
- Endometrioid carcinomas are seen to be associated in patients with endometriosis and endometrial carcinoma of the uterus.
- Germ cell tumors of malignant variety are usually seen in the young patients less than 20 years of age. These secrete human chorionic gonadotropin (hCG) and alpha-fetoprotein (AFP) and are thus the tumor markers for them. Most common of these is dysgerminomas and seen in association with gonadal dysgenesis. Unilateral oophorectomy is done in these cases followed by chemotherapy with good prognosis. Immature teratoma is the malignant counterpart of dermoid cyst. It is a rapidly growing tumor and produces painful symptomatology due to hemorrhage and necrosis. Other less common types are embryonal cell carcinomas, mixed germ cell tumors, and endodermal sinus tumors (Fig. 9.3).

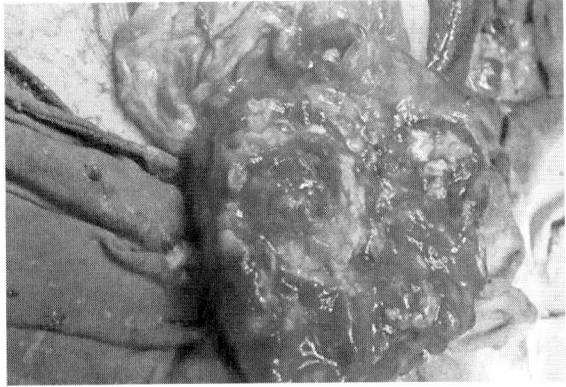

Fig. 9.3: Rare presentation of ruptured malignant germ cell tumor in a 12-year-old girl.
(For Color Version, See Color Plate 2)

- Granulosa cell tumors may lead to endometrial hyperplasia and endometrial carcinomas, due to its estrogen releasing property. In patients who have completed their family, total hysterectomy with bilateral salpingo-oophorectomy along with staging is done. Sertoli-Leydig cell tumor, on the other hand, produces virilizing symptoms in patients with adnexal mass.
- Krukenberg's tumor is the description of the metastasis to bilateral ovaries, primary lesion being gastrointestinal tumors and breast carcinomas.

A special mention about borderline ovarian tumors: Usually, it is seen in the age group of 30–50 years. These tumors may contain histological evidence of intraepithelial neoplasm, and the treatment of these tumors has to be individualized as per the patient.

APPROACH TO THE PATIENT WITH OVARIAN CYST

History and Examination

The approach to a patient presenting with ovarian cyst begins with a thorough history including the age and parity of the patient, presenting complaints, its onset and rate of progression taking especially into consideration the risk factors for malignancy. The symptoms in patients with ovarian malignancy are usually vague and include persistent abdominal or pelvic pain, early satiety, abdominal fullness, increased urinary frequency, and urgency as they usually present in later stage and early stage of ovarian malignancies are asymptomatic. Here, thus lies the importance of correct diagnosis and as early as possible. Rarely, one finds the patients presenting with acute presentation, where the possibility of torsion, rupture, or hemorrhage in the ovarian mass should be expected. *The family history of breast and ovarian malignancy* is important as well, more so when first-degree relative is affected. If the patient or her relative is a known carrier of *BRCA1*, *BRCA2*, mismatch repair gene mutation, more so the risk of malignancy increases.

The *physical examination* is equally important. The abdominal examination accompanied by vaginal and rectal examination adds to the knowledge of the physician, although it has a poor sensitivity of 15–51%. The findings like feeling of an irregular fixed, solid mass; the mass which is bilateral associated with ascites and generalized lymphadenopathy is suggestive of ovarian malignancy.

Imaging Modality

Imaging is most important in diagnosing the exact nature of the mass and ultrasonography with Doppler flows is one of the best modality available that helps in knowing the character of the mass and thus planning further management. Transvaginal ultrasonography along with transabdominal ultrasound gives better details in cases of large ovarian masses or presence of extraovarian disease. Ultrasound Doppler improves the sensitivity of detection of these masses especially in cases of complex cysts. In patients presenting with acute abdomen, the best modality of imaging is again ultrasound with Doppler flows to rule out torsion. Even advanced imaging modalities like computed tomography (CT) scan and magnetic resonance imaging (MRI) are required in cases of complex ovarian cysts. CT scan should not be used as a primary modality for the assessment of ovarian cysts in view of its low specificity, the use of ionizing radiation and high cost. Even, MRI is used when the nature of the cyst cannot be clearly defined with the help of an ultrasound. So, if from clinical and radiological assessment possibility of malignant disease cannot be excluded, timely referral to gynecological oncology multidisciplinary team is appropriate.

Tumor Markers

Next step is the measurement of serum levels of ovarian markers, most important being *CA 125* levels. Value more than 35 IU/mL is considered significant, but in postmenopausal women, the threshold decreases. It is a primary measure of epithelial ovarian malignancy and is raised in 50% of early stage disease. It is also seen to be raised in benign conditions like pelvic infections, endometriosis, adenomyosis, and fibroids and also in nongynecological conditions like hepatitis, ascites, pancreatitis, and cancers with peritoneal spread like breast and colon. Thus, it is of relatively less value in premenopausal women as compared to postmenopausal women is assessing ovarian masses. Also, single elevated value is of little significance as compared to progressively increasing levels of CA 125 level, where it is more suggestive of possibility of malignancy. Thus, CA 125 level is not very sensitive and specific marker, but is very helpful in prognostication and follow-up of the patient. Other markers like *lactate dehydrogenase (LDH), AFP,* and *beta-hCG* should be measured in all patients of age less than 40 years presenting with complex mass on ultrasound because of the possibility of germ cell tumors. *HE-4* (human epididymis) is yet another marker found to be of relevance in cases of ovarian mass and found to more sensitive and specific than CA 125.

At present, Risk Malignancy Index (RMI) is the most commonly used index to assess the nature of ovarian cyst in a patient. RMI is simple to use and easily reproducible.

$$RMI = U \times M \times CA125$$

- The ultrasound result is scored 1 point each for each of the following characteristics: multilocular cyst, solid areas, bilateral, metastasis, and ascites. U = 0 for none such features, 1 for one feature and 3 for more than one such features on ultrasound.
- M = 1 for premenopausal and 3 for postmenopausal females.
- CA 125 levels measured in IU/mL (Table 9.3).

Table 9.3: Risk malignancy index (RMI) and its association with the risk of malignancy.

RMI	Risk of malignancy
<25	3%
25–250	20%
>250	75%

Table 9.4: International Ovarian Tumor Analysis (IOTA) group ultrasound rules to classify masses as benign or malignant.

B-rule	M-rule
Unilocular cyst	Irregular solid tumor
Presence of solid components where large solid components are <7 mm	Ascites
Presence of acoustic shadowing	At least four papillary structure
Smooth multilocular tumor with largest diameter <100 mm	Irregular multilocular solid tumor with largest diameter >100 mm
No blood flows	Very strong blood flows

The RMI value greater than 200 has a sensitivity of 78% and a specificity of 87%, and so a need to refer the patient to gynecology oncology center.

The next comes the IOTA (International Ovarian Tumor Analysis), which involves use of ultrasound in differentiating benign from malignant ovarian masses (Table 9.4).

So, patient having any of the M-rules on ultrasound findings should be referred to gynecology oncology center.

Some of the recent indices are *ROMA* and *OVA1*. ROMA is a quantitative test using CA 125 levels, HE-4, and menopausal status to calculate the risk of ovarian cancer. A numerical score is calculated based on algorithm equation calculation with cut off value of 2.27 representing high risk of malignancy. It is helpful in distinguishing epithelial ovarian cancer from benign ovarian cysts. The other modality is OVA1. It measures five serum proteins that are CA1 25, transthyretin, apolipoprotein A1, beta-2 glycoprotein, and transferrin and combining them into numerical score. This uses special software and specific assays of the markers and value more than 4.4 is indicative of high risk of malignancy, especially in postmenopausal woman.

About 10% of woman will have some of the surgery during their life time for presence of ovarian cysts. 1:1,000 cysts in premenopausal women are malignant and this increases to 5:1,000 at the age of 50 years. Preoperative differentiation between benign and malignant is usually difficult, in spite of all the advances. So, the aim should be to optimize the management of the patient as per the clinical, radiological, and biochemical findings and decrease patient's morbidity by planning conservative management whenever possible and use of minimally invasive surgery where appropriate.

So, in a *premenopausal patient* presenting with an asymptomatic cyst should be followed up according to the size as per latent RCOG (Royal College of Obstetricians and Gynecologists) guidelines.

- An asymptomatic cyst, unilocular and simple on ultrasound of less than 5 cm, does not require a follow-up even as it is seen to resolve with time, usually within 3 menstrual cycles.
- A cyst of size 5–7 cm, simple, unilocular, and belonging to the B-rule category on ultrasound, requires follow-up on yearly basis.
- A simple cyst of more than 7 cm should be considered for further extensive workup to decipher its nature and plan surgical management accordingly.
- Persisting ovarian cyst or that increasing in size requires surgical management.

In *postmenopausal woman*:
- An asymptomatic cyst of less than 5 cm, with normal CA 125 levels, requires conservative approach with follow-up every 4–6 months.
- A size of more than 5 cm requires surgical management.

The use of hormonal pills is equivalent to not using any drug for a patient planned to be on conservative management for the ovarian cyst. So, the need to give or omit should be weighed by the treating physician.

All symptomatic masses, having M-rule on ultrasound, and highlighting endometriomas of size more than 3 cm require surgical management. Mainly in the form of laparoscopic evaluation and proceed.

The mode of surgery to a great extent depends on the place of surgery and the expertise of the surgeon. Laparoscopic route is presumed to be the best, in terms of its minimal access, lower postoperative morbidity, and shorter recovery time. It is mandatory to avoid spillage of contents, as it can upstage a malignant disease, if existing and also can lead to chemical peritonitis as in case of dermoid cysts. All masses should be removed in an endobag. The aim should be to preserve the ovary whenever possible. In patients, who are suspected to be in advanced stage of ovarian malignancy or very large ovarian masses or with no laparoscopic expertise available, it is better to go for staging laparotomy followed by total abdominal hysterectomy with bilateral salpingo-oophorectomy and omentectomy with lymphadenectomy.

In patients presenting with acute abdomen due to ovarian torsion should be best managed laparoscopically as early as possible. Conservative management with detorsion is highly recommended irrespective of the appearance of the ovary. Involvement of the fallopian tube in the torsion of

Table 9.5: Referral guidelines for a newly diagnosed pelvic mass [American College of Obstetricians and Gynecologists (ACOG) practice guidelines].

Premenopausal women (younger than 50 years)	<ul><li>Family history of breast or ovarian malignancy in first-degree relative</li><li>CA 125 levels greater than 200 IU/mL</li><li>Ascites</li><li>Evidence of abdominal or distant metastasis</li></ul>
Postmenopausal women (more than 50 years old)	<ul><li>Family history of breast or ovarian malignancy in first-degree relative</li><li>CA 125 levels greater than 35 IU/mL</li><li>Ascites</li><li>Evidence of abdominal or distant metastasis</li><li>Nodular fixed mass</li></ul>

the adnexa may damage the tube significantly, which may then need to be surgically removed (Table 9.5).

CONCLUSION

So, to conclude any patient, be it premenopausal or postmenopausal with ovarian cyst should be thoroughly evaluated. It includes thorough history taking, physical examination, appropriate imaging and tumor markers to evaluate the nature of the ovarian cyst. The management of the ovarian cysts should be individualized, including the mode and the extent of the surgery to optimize patient outcome.

SUGGESTED READING

1. American College of Obstetrics and Gynecologists. Management of adnexal masses. ACOG Practice Bulletin No. 83. Obstet Gynecol. 2007;110(1):201-14.
2. Royal Collage of Obstetrician and Gynaecologists. (2011). Management of suspected ovarian masses in premenopausal women. Green top guidelines No. 62. [online] Available from https://www.rcog.org.uk/globalassets/documents/guidelines/gtg_62.pdf. [Accessed November, 2018].
3. Royal Collage of Obstetrician and Gynaecologists. (2016). The management of ovarian cysts in postmenopausal women. Green top guidelines No. 34. [online] Available from https://www.rcog.org.uk/en/guidelines-research-services/guidelines/gtg34/. [Accessed November, 2018].

CHAPTER 10

Pelvic Inflammatory Disease

Kanwal Gujral

INTRODUCTION

Pelvic inflammatory disease (PID) is an acute or subclinical infection of upper reproductive tract—the uterus, fallopian tubes and the ovaries. All organs may be involved, but organ of importance is fallopian tube. Hence, another diagnosis given to PID is acute salpingitis. About 85% of PID is a sexually transmitted infection, the two most common causative organisms being *Neisseria gonorrhoeae* and *Chlamydia trachomatis*. Bacterial vaginosis occasionally can also lead to PID. Fifteen percent of PID is due to nonsexually transmitted pathogens, which could be a postoperative infection, trauma-related pelvic infection, procedure related infection (dilation curettage, abortions, etc.) or secondary to another infection like appendicitis. Long-term sequelae associated with PID are infertility, chronic pelvic pain and ectopic pregnancy.

RISK FACTORS FOR PELVIC INFLAMMATORY DISEASE

- Young age
- Multiple sexual partners, recent new partner
- Sexually transmitted disease (STD) in partner
- Drug addicts
- Previous history of PID
- Recent instrumentation
- Low socioeconomic status
- Pregnancy.

Note: Barrier contraception protects against PID, condom being the most effective one.

ACUTE PELVIC INFLAMMATORY DISEASE

Pathogenesis and Microbiology

Vaginal flora of healthy normal women contains potentially pathogenic organism which lie in a dormant condition. *Lactobacillus* species is a nonpathogenic organism, abundantly present in vagina. Under unfavorable conditions, there is an imbalance between pathogens and the protective *Lactobacilli* former exceeding the later, allowing ascent of pathogen into upper genital tract which can cause PID. Endocervical canal mucus plug acts as a protective barrier. When this barrier is disrupted, organisms can ascend and cause infection of endocervix, endometrium, inner lining of fallopian tube (the endosalpinx) ovarian cortex and finally the pelvic peritoneum. The resultant effects are endocervicitis, endometritis, acute salpingitis, oophoritis, tubo-ovarian masses or tubo-ovarian abscess, pelvic peritonitis and in the event of a leaking or ruptured abscess, general peritonitis and pyoperitoneum. Inflammation of the liver capsule and its peritoneal surface can also occur. This is referred to as perihepatitis or Fitz-Hugs-Curtis syndrome and is seen in 10% of the cases.

It is important to remember that pulmonary tuberculosis can also cause salpingitis and endometritis by blood-borne spread but ascension may also be a possible route.

Sexually transmitted pathogens causing PID are *Neisseria gonorrhoeae* and *Chlamydia trachomatis*, while nonsexually transmitted pathogens are *Streptococci, Staphylococci, Enterobacters* (*Klebsiella, Escherichia coli* and *Proteus*), *Haemophilus, Bacteroides, Peptostreptococcus* and some anaerobes. Recent evidence from United Kingdom (UK) has linked *Mycoplasma genitalium* to sexually transmitted infection. Rarely Actinomycete in long-term intrauterine device users can be a causative organism.

Note: It is important to remember that in a vast majority of PID cases, infection is polymicrobial in nature.

Clinical Diagnosis

Recent onset of pain in lower abdomen is the cardinal presenting symptom usually following a sexual contact. Pain shortly after menstruation is also suggestive.

Florid discharge, abnormal uterine bleeding which is either postcoital, intermenstrual or prolonged, urinary frequency, fever, chills, anorexia, nausea, vomiting, diarrhea are other presenting symptoms.

Per abdomen examination: Most women have tender iliac fossa or tender lower abdomen. Rigidity or rebound tenderness may or may not be present. If all quadrants of abdomen are tender, then rupture of tubo-ovarian (TO) abscess should be suspected.

Per speculum and bimanual pelvic examination: Purulent discharge from cervix is often seen. Cervical motion tenderness, uterine, forniceal tenderness is seen in acute phase. Later pelvic masses can be felt. Fluctuating mass in pouch of Douglas is a sign of pelvic abscess. Clinical diagnosis is correct in 65–90% of cases.

Laboratory Diagnosis

- Leukocytosis more than 12,000/cubic mm, raised erythrocyte sedimentation rate (ESR) more than or equal to 40 mm/h, C-reactive protein (CRP) more than 60 mg/L.
- Saline microscopy of vaginal discharge—15–20 WBC/hpf or white blood cells (WBCs) more than epithelial cells.
- Gram-staining of cervical discharge—positive Gram stain is suggestive of *Neisseria gonorrhoeae*.
- Nucleic acid amplification test (NAAT)—for *Chlamydia trachomatis* and *N. gonorrhoeae*.

Other recommended laboratory tests: Serology of syphilis, screening for hepatitis B, human immunodeficiency virus (HIV) and β-human chorionic gonadotropin (β-hCG) test to rule out pregnancy. In Indian scenario, it is wise to rule out underlying tubercular infection.

Imaging

Ultrasonography

Thick, distended fallopian tubes, tender fallopian tubes are important diagnostic features in the initial phases. Cogwheel appearance on cross section of fallopian tube may also be seen. Fluid in pouch of Douglas (POD) aids to diagnosis. In the event of endometritis being present, fluid or gas in endometrial cavity, thick heterogeneous endometrial lining may also be seen. Doppler ultrasound may show increased blood flow, a sign of acute salpingitis.

Tubo-ovarian mass or abscess will depict a complex multiloculated thick-walled structure with multiple fluid levels or internal echoes (Figs. 10.1A and B).

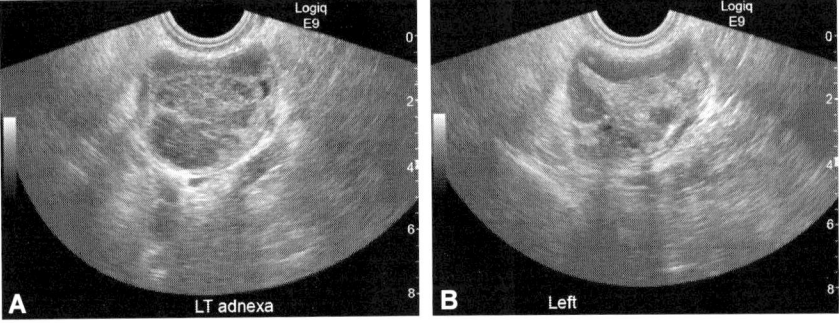

Figs. 10.1A and B: Ultrasound images tubo-ovarian (TO) mass.

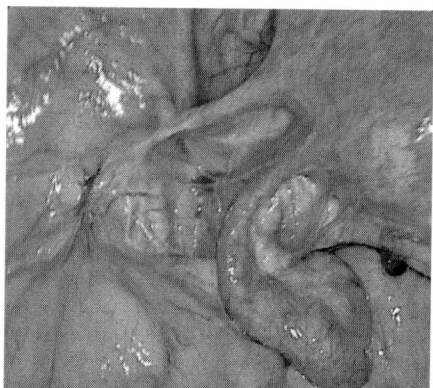

Fig. 10.2: Laparoscopy picture tubo-ovarian adhesions.
(For Color Version, See Color Plate 3)

Computed Tomography or Magnetic Resonance Imaging

These imaging modalities can delineate to masses with precision but are generally used to exclude alternate diagnosis when presentation is atypical or severe.

Laparoscopy

It has high specificity in diagnosing PID, but has low sensitivity. Tubal edema, erythema, abnormal fimbria, purulent exudate from fimbria and fluid in cul-de-sac are hallmark signs of acute PID. Positive bacteriology of fluid further strengthens the diagnosis. Laparoscopy is an invasive procedure, therefore it is recommended as a part of diagnostic workup if there is no improvement after 72 hours of treatment or an alternate diagnosis is suspected or clinical findings and imaging studies are inconclusive or an intervention is planned along with (Fig. 10.2).

Endometrial Biopsy

Endometrial biopsy can detect endometritis by depicting inflammatory cells but is not routinely recommended.

Generally a temperature more than 38°C, abnormal cervical discharge, clinical findings and a positive saline microscopy is sufficient to diagnose acute PID. A low threshold for suspecting PID should be the norm.

A normal cervical discharge, no WBC on saline microscopy, predominantly urinary or gastrointestinal (GI) symptoms nearly rules out PID. It is extremely important to rule out ectopic pregnancy in a young woman.

Treatment

Since majority of PIDs are polymicrobial in nature, broad-spectrum antibiotic coverage is recommended as an initial treatment, whether treated as an inpatient or outpatient.

Indications for Inpatient Treatment
- Adolescent girls.
- Drug addicts.
- Severe clinical illness—high-grade fever, gastrointestinal (GI) symptoms such as nausea, vomiting, abdominal pain, suspected abscess and generalized peritonitis.
- Failed outpatient therapy, intolerance to oral therapy, noncompliance.
- Uncertain diagnosis or suspected alternate diagnosis.
- Need for surgical intervention.
- Pregnancy.

Acute Pelvic Inflammatory Disease: Inpatient Therapy
First-line parenteral antibiotic therapy:
- *Regimen 1*: Cefoxitin 2 g IV 6 hourly or cefotetan 2 g IV 12 hourly
  - Doxycycline 100 mg IV or oral 12 hourly × 14 days.
- *Regimen 2*: Clindamycin 900 mg IV 8 hourly plus
  - Gentamycin loading dose 2 mg/kg followed by maintenance dose of 1.5 mg/kg
  - Single dose of gentamycin 2–7 mg/kg/day can be an alternative.
- Few other used regimens are:
  - Levofloxacin 500 mg IV daily or ofloxacin 400 mg IV 12 hourly with or without metronidazole 500 mg IV 8 hourly
  - Combination of ampicillin-sulbactam 3 g IV 6 hourly along with doxycycline 100 mg 12 hourly IV or orally.
- Intravenous antibiotics should be continued for a period of 48–72 hours. A good clinical improvement is usually seen during this period. After this a switch to oral therapy can be done. Doxycycline therapy should be continued for 14 days.
- Patients with pelvic abscess should receive clindamycin 450 mg orally 6 hourly or metronidazole 500 mg 8 hourly for 14 days along with doxycycline.
- Antiemetics, antipyretics, IV hydration, fluid and electrolyte balance is strongly recommended along with antibiotic therapy.

Outpatient Therapy
Mild to moderate PIDs can be treated safely on an outpatient basis. Centers for Disease Control and Prevention (CDC) 2015 recommends any of the following regimens:
- Ceftriaxone 250 mg (IM) intramuscularly single dose along with doxycycline 100 mg twice daily for 14 days with or without metronidazole 500 mg twice daily for 14 days.
- Cefoxitin 2 g IM single dose along with a single dose of probenecid 1 g oral. Doxycycline 100 mg twice daily for 14 days with or without metronidazole 500 mg twice daily for 14 days should be given in addition.

- Cefotaxime 1 g IM single dose or ceftizoxime 1 g IM single dose plus doxycycline with or without metronidazole as above.
- Azithromycin has a long half-life and a good intracellular concentration besides easy dosing schedule. One trial has compared a combination of single IM injection of ceftriaxone and doxycycline with combination of azithromycin 1 g weekly for 4 weeks plus doxycycline for 14 days with equal response rate.

Note: Patients treated for PID on outpatient basis must be evaluated in 48–72 hours to see the response and be admitted in case of no improvement within 72 hours.

Follow-up

- Immunization against hepatitis B virus (HBV), human papillomavirus (HPV) is recommended if women have not been vaccinated earlier.
- Barrier contraception is strongly recommended. Condoms have the highest protection rate. Progesterone based contraception also offer protection by making cervical mucus thick.
- Screening and treating the partner is mandatory.

Treatment Controversies

- Centers for Disease Control and Prevention guidelines 2007 have indicated that fluoroquinolones are no longer recommended as a therapy for PID if *Gonococcus* is proven or suspected.
- Also there is lack of consensus on the role of routine anaerobic coverage. Some experts suggest that anaerobic coverage with metronidazole should be given if the infection is severe or there is presence of tubo-ovarian mass.

Inpatient Treatment versus Outpatient Treatment

Pelvic Inflammation Disease Evaluation Clinical Health (PEACH) trial has indicated similar efficacy in terms of short-term clinical outcome, microbiological outcome and long-term reproductive outcomes like chronic pelvic pain, ectopic pregnancy in women with mild to moderate PID whether treatment is on inpatient or outpatient basis.

Surgical Intervention

Patients with pelvic abscess, tubo-ovarian abscess not responding to antimicrobial therapy by 72 hours or if there is general peritonitis, are candidates for surgical intervention. Pelvic abscess can be drained from vagina but tubo-ovarian abscess needs an abdominal approach preferably by laparoscopy. Drainage of TO abscess, removal of debris through peritoneal lavage and postoperative drain placement is key to successful surgical treatment.

Silent Pelvic Inflammatory Disease

This results from multiple or low grade infection, usually after incomplete treatment. The diagnosis is often given to women who present with tubal factor infertility. There is often a history of previous PID. At laparoscopy or laparotomy common encountered findings are paratubal adhesions, ovarian adhesions, thickened tubes, blocked tubes or hydrosalpinx.

Long-term Sequelae of Pelvic Inflammatory Disease

Sequelae include infertility (15-20%), chronic pelvic pain (30%), recurrent PID (15-20%), tubal pregnancy (7-8%). A weak link between previous PID and ovarian cancer has been reported.

CONCLUSION

- Pelvic inflammatory disease is an acute or subclinical infection of upper reproductive tract—the uterus, fallopian tubes and the ovaries.
- Approximately 85% of infections are sexually transmitted whereas 15% are nonsexually transmitted.
- Infection most often is polymicrobial in nature.
- Diagnosis is usually clinical and is correct in 65-90% of the cases.
- Further diagnostic workup includes saline microscopy of vaginal discharge, culture of specific organisms and ultrasonography.
- Computed tomography and MRI are generally used to exclude other causes.
- Laparoscopy is recommended as a part of diagnostic workup if imaging studies are inconclusive or there is no improvement within 72 hours of medical treatment.
- Majority of the patients can be managed as outpatients.
- Indications for hospitalization include severe clinical illness, noncompliant patients, adolescent girls, uncertain diagnosis or a need for surgical intervention.
- Center for Disease Control and Prevention has outlined multiple treatment regimens with proven efficacy both for inpatients and outpatients.
- Follow-up includes vaccination against HBV, HPV and screening and treatment of partner.
- Barrier contraception offers protection against PID.
- Long-term sequelae are infertility, chronic pelvic pain and ectopic pregnancy.

SUGGESTED READING

1. Centers for Disease Control and Prevention (CDC). Update to CDC's sexually transmitted diseases treatment guidelines, 2006: fluoroquinolones no longer recommended for treatment of gonococcal infections. MMWR Morb Mortal Wkly Rep. 2007;56(14):332-6.

2. Ness RB, Soper DE, Holly RL, et al. Effectiveness of inpatient and outpatient treatment strategies for women with pelvic inflammatory disease: results from the Pelvic Inflammatory Disease Evaluation and Clinical Health (PEACH) Randomized Trial. Am J Obstet Gynecol. 2002;186(5):929-37.
3. Ross JDC, Mc Carthy J. (2011). UK National Guideline for Management of Pelvic Inflammatory Disease (BASHH) JD. Ross and G McCarthy. 2011. http://www.bashh.org/guidelines.
4. Walker CK, Wiesenfeld HC. Antibiotic therapy for acute pelvic inflammatory disease: the 2006 centers for Disease Control and Prevention sexually transmitted disease treatment guidelines. Clin Infect Dis. 2007;44(Suppl 3):S111-22.
5. Workowski KA, Bolan GA, Centers for Disease Control and Prevention. Sexually transmitted diseases treatment guideline, 2015. MMWR Recomm Rep. 2015;64(RR-03):1-137.

CHAPTER

11

The Enigma of Polycystic Ovarian Syndrome

Ruma Satwik

INTRODUCTION

Polycystic ovarian syndrome (PCOS) is a condition as old as mankind. The earliest record exists in the writings of Hippocrates (460-377 BC), who linked reduced frequency of menstruation to infertility. Subsequently Soranus (98-138 AD) identified women who had reduced frequency of menstruation as the ones with a rather "robust, mannish" appearance. It was not until 1935 that Irving Freiler Stein (1887-1976) and Michael Leo Leventhal (1901-1971) linked the symptoms of oligoovulation, hirsutism, obesity and infertility with ovarian morphology and coined the term polycystic ovaries. They described ovarian wedge resection as a cure for this condition. The etiopathogenesis and manifestations of this condition remained an enigma to the reproductive physicians for several years. This is reflected in the several terms that were coined to describe it: Stein-Leventhal syndrome, polycystic ovarian disease or disorder, hyperandrogenic chronic anovulation, functional ovary androgenism, sclerotic polycystic ovary syndrome, syndrome X and ovarian dysmetabolic syndrome.

DEFINITION AND DIAGNOSIS

The current definition of PCOS employs various combinations of three clinical criteria—ovulatory disturbance, androgen excess and polycystic ovarian morphology, after ruling out other causes of androgen excess. Previous criteria like insulin resistance, altered follicle stimulating hormone (FSH) or luteinizing hormone (LH) ratio, obesity, etc. may be associated features but no longer necessary for defining the syndrome (Box 11.1).

Three definitions of PCOS are currently in use:
1. Rotterdam's European Society of Human Reproduction and Embryology (ESHRE) and American Society for Reproductive Medicine (ASRM)-PCOS working group definition (2003).
2. National Institute of Health definition (1990).
3. Androgen Excess Society Definition (2006).

> **Box 11.1:** Criteria for defining polycystic ovarian syndrome (PCOS).
>
> - Ovulatory disturbance (OD)
>   - Anovulation, oligoovulation
>   - Androgen excess (AE)
> - *Biochemical*: High concentration of total or free testosterone, high free androgen index
> - *Clinical*: Hirsutism, acne
>   - Polycystic ovarian morphology (PCOM)
>   - Ovarian volume >10 cc^3
>   - Antral follicle count (AFC) ≥ 12 in one or both ovaries.

> **Box 11.2:** Polycystic ovarian syndrome (PCOS) definitions by different criteria.
>
> | | National Institute of Health (NIH) 1990 | Rotterdam's 2003 | Androgen excess society 2006 |
> | --- | --- | --- | --- |
> | Ovulatory disturbance | + | ± | ± |
> | Androgen excess | + | ± | + |
> | Polycystic appearance | | ± | ± |

Rotterdam's (2003) definition of PCOS requires any two out of three criteria to be present. It takes a liberal view in defining the syndrome and allows for the existence of four PCOS phenotypes: OD + AE, OD + PCOM, AE + PCOM, OD + AE + PCOM.

National Institute of Health (1990) defines it as the presence of both ovulatory disturbance and androgen excess. It is a stricter definition and recognizes only the OD + AE phenotype as having PCOS. It disregards ovarian morphology completely.

Androgen excess society (2006) seeks to achieve a middle ground between the two. It mandates the presence of androgen excess along with the presence of either ovulatory disturbance or polycystic appearance of ovaries to define PCOS. Thus it allows for three phenotypes, AE + OD, AE + PCOM, AE + OD + PCOM (Box 11.2).

All the three definitions require other causes of androgen excess to be ruled out such as:
- Exogenous androgen intake
- Ovarian or adrenal tumors
- Congenital adrenal hyperplasia
- Cushing's syndrome.

CRITERIA IN ADOLESCENCE

Polycystic ovarian syndrome has its beginnings in fetal life and starts to manifest as early as the initial years of adolescence. However, it is difficult

> **Box 11.3:** Criteria for polycystic ovarian syndrome (PCOS) diagnosis in adolescence.
>
> Criteria for PCOS diagnosis in adolescence
>
> All three should be present:
> 1. Menstrual irregularity persisting beyond 2 years of menarche
> 2. Hyperandrogenemia rather than clinical hyperandrogenism
> 3. Ovarian volume >10 cm³ rather than AFC >12.
>
> Identify groups at risk but be cautious about pronouncing the diagnosis.

to ascertain at this stage whether ovulatory disturbance or signs of androgen excess is due to the not yet fully matured hypothalamic-pituitary-ovarian (HPO) or hypothalamic-pituitary-adrenal (HPA) axes or due to PCOS. Hence, the criteria for diagnosing PCOS in adolescence are stricter as deemed by the 2010 ESHRE-ASRM consensus meet (Box 11.3).

Prevalence

Polycystic ovarian syndrome is the most common endocrine disorder in women. Prevalence between 6% by NIH criteria and 10–15% by Rotterdam's criteria has been reported amongst reproductive age women, in literature. The reported incidence amongst Indians is 9–10%. The predominant phenotypic characteristics vary with ethnicity. Oriental women have a lower incidence of hirsutism and higher incidence of PCOM. Mediterranean women show higher degree of hirsutism. Indian PCOS women are more likely to be obese with insulin resistance.

Etiology

Polycystic ovarian syndrome has a multifactorial etiology. Its manifestations are now known to occur as an end interaction between three primary factors—a genetic predisposition, intrauterine fetal programming and extrauterine aggravation due to lifestyle.

Genetic Predisposition

Number of candidate genes implicated in PCOS is increasing. Genetic abnormalities in androgen steroidogenesis and in insulin action have been detected in PCOS patients like mutations in genes coding for sex-hormone-binding globulin (SHBG), Cytochrome P450-17 (CYP17), hydroxylase/17, 20 lyase enzyme, androgen receptor, insulin and insulin receptor. But no single gene has been shown a consistent link to PCOS. It is now understood to be a polygenic condition requiring combinations of different genes to explain heterogeneity. The current genetic studies have failed to identify specific gene or genes, with clear clinical significance and practically do not take our clinical approach any further from the significant initial observation that a positive family history is common in women with PCOS.

Intrauterine Conditioning

Prenatal androgen exposure: Fetal genes can be silenced or overexpressed by the environment it encounters in its intrauterine sojourn. It has been known for some years now that maternal androgen excess at specific time during pregnancy could lead to a PCOS like picture in the exposed female offspring after puberty. In experimental models that created an environment of prenatal androgen excess by administering exogenous androgens to pregnant rhesus monkeys, it was seen that the female offspring developed PCOS-like abnormalities later in life, including a combination of reproductive and metabolic abnormalities. LH in the affected offspring increased postnatally, possibly due to a reduction in the ability of gonadotropin-releasing hormone (GnRH) releasing neurons to respond to the negative feedback action of sex steroids.

This intrauterine conditioning of the GnRH pulse generator due to high androgens, have been incriminated in the mechanism of PCOS in women born to PCOS mothers, rather than a direct inheritance of multiple genes.

The adipose tissue expandability theory: Whenever an individual is in positive energy balance caused by excessive calorie intake, the surplus energy gets stored in the form of lipids in adipose tissues. This phenomenon of lipid storage in adipose cells occurs through the process of adipose tissue expansion. All individuals possess a maximum capacity for adipose expansion. Once the adipose tissue expansion limit is reached, adipose tissue ceases to store energy efficiently and lipids begin to accumulate in other tissues.

Adipose tissue expandability is determined by both genetic and intrauterine factors. In fetuses with intrauterine malnutrition, both hypoplasia and hypotrophy of adipose tissue exists. Such individuals who have suffered intrauterine malnutrition quickly exhaust their capacity to expand subcutaneous adipose tissue. Even small energy excesses that now cannot be accommodated in their hypoplastic adipose tissue, easily spill to visceral tissue like that of abdominal wall, pancreas, liver and heart. This visceral fat is resistant to insulin action. Insulin resistance and hyperinsulinemia can then cause a picture of ovarian hyperandrogenism and anovulation.

Lifestyle

What we eat and drink and how we live can affect the severity of manifestations of PCOS. A high carbohydrate, high sugar, low fiber diet aggravates the metabolic disorder. Sedentary lifestyles lead to energy surplus and consequent storage as fat. Smoking, stress, long working hours and sleep deprivation could exacerbate the HPO axis dysfunction (Flowchart 11.1).

Pathogenesis

How does hyperandrogenemia lead to the manifestations of PCOS? High local levels of ovarian androgens obstruct folliculogenesis at the mid-antral

Flowchart 11.1: Etiopathogenesis of polycystic ovarian syndrome (PCOS).

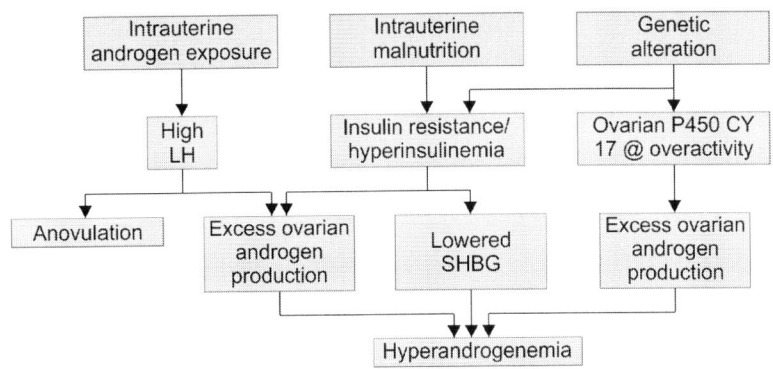

(LH: luteinizing hormone; SHBG: sex-hormone-binding globulin gene).

stage, prevent apoptosis of follicles, causing more and more mid-antral follicles to accumulate in the polycystic ovary that are neither growing nor dying, waiting for a rising FSH signal to rescue them. This rise in FSH that normally begins with menstruation is lacking in PCOS women owing to a steady anovulatory signal from the hypothalamus. Thus the characteristic appearance of a polycystic ovary containing numerous follicles suspended in the 2–8 mm stage develops.

Also, androgens in peripheral fat get converted to estrogens particularly estrone. This by negative feedback on the hypothalamus causes high frequency, low amplitude secretion of GnRH, which favors LH and inhibits FSH release. This alters the FSH-LH ratio enough to act in tandem with locally increased androgens to stop folliculogenesis and ovulation.

Clinical Features: Presentation, Examination and Investigations

The spectrum of the disorder varies according to age with menstrual irregularity and acne being the predominant complaint in young adolescents, infertility and hirsutism afflicting women in reproductive years and metabolic syndrome aggravated by obesity being the presenting symptom in perimenopausal women (Fig. 11.1).

Polycystic ovarian syndrome can present with a range of abnormalities relating to menstruation, although a minority of them, comprising not more than 5% of the total, may continue to be eumenorrheic. The menstrual abnormalities seen in the order of decreasing frequency are oligomenorrhea, secondary amenorrhea, polymenorrhea; metrorrhagia and hypomenorrhea. The greater the menstrual irregularity, the more severe is the PCOS phenotype. Menstrual cycles in women with PCOS may become more regular later in life.

Women with oligomenorrhea or amenorrhea have about a 90% chance of being diagnosed with PCOS, the other causes being hypothyroidism,

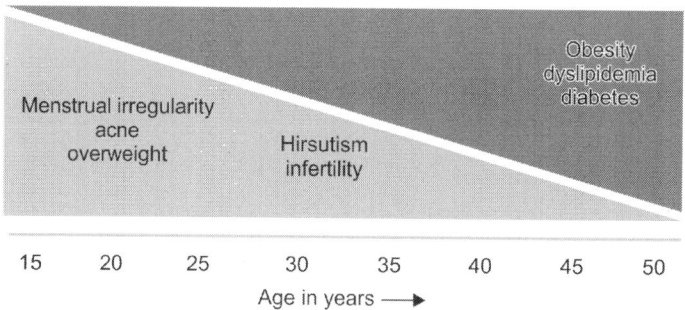

Fig. 11.1: Age-wise manifestation of polycystic ovarian syndrome (PCOS).

hyperprolactinemia, hypogonadotropic-hypogonadism, adrenal disorders and premature ovarian failure which need to be ruled out by careful history, examination and investigations.

Hyperandrogenemia of PCOS manifests as hirsutism and acne. Central balding, clitoromegaly and hoarseness of voice are usually not associated with PCOS and are more likely to be seen in women with androgen producing tumors. Hirsutism is the presence of coarse hair in androgenic areas in women. It is objectively assessed by Ferriman-Gallwey scoring system. This system assigns a score of 0 to 4 to the severity of hirsutism based on coarseness, density and pigmentation in each of the nine areas assessed, namely chin, upper lip, lower lip, chest, upper abdomen, lower abdomen, thighs, upper back and lower back. A maximum score of 36 and a minimum of 0 could be assigned. Scores above 8 generally denote significant hirsutism in Indian population.

Hyperandrogenemia is a defining feature of PCOS. The most common biochemical abnormality causing hyperandrogenemia is high free testosterone levels. Dehydroepiandrosterone (DHEA) may be elevated in 5% of women with PCOS. The other androgens like; total testosterone, and androstenedione and dihydrotestosterone show elevations infrequently.

Luteinizing hormone or FSH ratio does not define PCOS. Although mean LH levels are higher in PCOS women than in non-PCOS women, the ratio does not always exceed 1 and could vary from anywhere between 3:1 and 1:2.

Features of associated metabolic syndrome might also be present like hypertension, hyperlipidemia and insulin resistance. Blood pressure more than 130/85 mm Hg has been labeled as hypertension. Hyperlipidemia in these women has been defined as high-density lipoproteins less than 50 mg% and triglycerides more than 150 mg%.

Features of insulin resistance are not present in all women with PCOS. Obesity acts as a significant add-on risk factor towards development of insulin resistance and its consequent complications. About 80% of obese PCOS women and 25% of lean PCOS women are found to be insulin resistant. Signs that the woman might be insulin resistant are central obesity, acanthosis nigricans, recurrent vulvovaginal candidiasis and an abnormal oral glucose tolerance test. Objective measures of central obesity are increased waist to hip ratio (> 0.85) and increased waist circumference of more than 88 cm [World Health Organization (WHO) standards in women]. Abdominal fat has been deemed to be metabolically healthy and more resistant to insulin action. Acanthosis nigricans is a purplish black discoloration of skin around the neck, armpits, groin and lower breast skin fold and is suggestive of hyperinsulinemia. Abnormal oral glucose tolerance test with fasting sugar more than 110 mg/dL and 2 hours. Postprandial sugar more than 140 mg/dL is also indicative of insulin resistance. Hyperglycemia increases vaginal lactic acid levels due to increased glucose breakdown. The increased acidic environment predisposes the woman to vulvovaginal candidiasis.

Endometrial hyperplasia (EH) and endometrial cancer (EC) has been associated with PCOS and is thought to be a result of persistent hyperestrogenemia unabated by progesterone action. However, the prevalence of EH and EC in well-characterized patients of hyperandrogenemia is not clearly known. In a Danish retrospective trans-sectional cohort study of all women referred to the health services between 1997 and 2008 as cases of PCOS with or without hirsutism, (n = 960) the incidence of EH was 1% and EC was 0.1%. This was not very different from controls. However, a Thai study of PCOS women with menstrual abnormalities undergoing endometrial aspiration (n = 57) found the incidence of EC-EH to be much higher at 19%. Perhaps it can be concluded, that those women with metrorrhagia, (heavy, prolonged and frequent bleeding) are more likely to have histological abnormalities than women with just oligomenorrhea, hypomenorrhea or amenorrhea.

A quick-look at salient points in examination, ultrasound and investigations are mentioned Boxes 11.4 to 11.6.

Box 11.4: Examination in polycystic ovary syndrome (PCOS).

- Height, weight, body mass index (BMI)
- Waist circumference
- Blood pressure
- Hirsutism
- Acne, hair balding
- Acanthosis nigricans
- Galactorrhea
- Thyroid swellings
- Vulvovaginal candidiasis

> **Box 11.5:** Ultrasound in polycystic ovary syndrome (PCOS).

- Ovarian volume: Length × width × depth × 0.623
- Antral follicle count: Early follicular phase
- Endometrial thickness and pattern: Early follicular phase
- Presence of ovarian or adrenal tumors.

> **Box 11.6:** Investigation in polycystic ovary syndrome (PCOS).

- Thyroid stimulating hormone (TSH), prolactin
- Serum testosterone free and total
- Free androgen index
- Dehydroepiandrosterone (DHEA) and dehydroepiandrosterone sulfate (DHEA-S)
- 17α-hydroxyprogesterone
- Oral glucose tolerance test (OGTT)
- Lipid profile.

MANAGEMENT

Lifestyle Modification

Polycystic ovarian syndrome is a genetic and epigenetic disorder that is conditioned by the modern day lifestyle. Only the latter is modifiable and the primary treatment in all women with PCOS across age-groups remains lifestyle modification. Delaying fertility therapy with preconception weight loss has helped in improving ovulation rates and live birth rates in obese PCOS women. This modification is aimed at reducing bodyweight to attain a healthy body mass index (BMI) of less than 23 kg/m². Even in those with ideal BMIs, abdominal obesity may be present. These women too benefit from a weight loss regime. Weight loss improves body composition, self-image, depression scores, lipid profiles, insulin resistance and menstrual irregularities.

Diet, exercise, pharmacotherapy and bariatric surgery are the four cardinal ways of weight loss.

Diet

It is the most effective and low cost way of losing weight. At least 5–10% weight loss should be the goal over three months. Lowering total calories helps. Altering dietary constituents to increase dietary fiber through fruits, vegetables, beans, etc. and lower high glycemic index food items like wheat, rice, sugar and sweetened beverages helps in achieving the target. Measures like fixed meal timings, avoiding snacking provide benefit too. In women with coexistent diabetes mellitus, smaller, more frequent meals (every 3–4 hours) help control blood glucose levels.

Exercise

Increasing activity through walking, jogging, cycling or climbing stairs helps in creating an energy deficit that achieves quicker weight loss. It also improves glucose uptake by muscles thus reducing hyperglycemia and hyperinsulinemia.

Pharmacotherapy

In women unable to control weight on diet alone, pharmacotherapy may be added under supervision of an expert.

- *Phentermine extended release (ER) topiramate*: An amphetamine analogue that enhances satiety by increasing hypothalamic noradrenaline levels. It should be started in low doses of 3.75 mg as a single dose in the morning. It may be increased up to 15 mg per day if no effect has been demonstrated despite 12 weeks of previous dose. Adverse effects include paresthesia, nausea, dizziness and constipation.
- *Orlistat*: It is an inhibitor of pancreatic and gastric lipase. It prevents fat digestion and absorption. It is given in doses of 60-120 mg thrice a day. Abdominal distention, steatorrhea, oxalate nephropathy are known side-effects.
- *Lorcaserin*: It is a selective serotonin agonist which stimulates generation of α-melanocortin to decrease food intake and enhance satiety. It is given in doses of 10 mg twice daily. Headache and hypoglycemia need to be watched out for.
- Phentermine-topiramate lowers weight by about 9-11 kg, lorcaserin by about 3-4 kg, and orlistat by about 2-3 kg after six to 12 months of treatment. Treatment is continued indefinitely in those who respond and stopped after 3-6 months in those who do not.

Surgery

Bariatric surgery is advised to morbidly obese women with BMI more than 40 kg/m^2 in whom the above methods have been ineffective. It is also advised to women with lower BMIs (between 35 and 40 kg/m^2) having coexistent morbidities like diabetes, hypertension, obstructive sleep apnea, etc. Surgeries work by two main mechanisms: either by restricting the gastric capacity (laparoscopic adjustable gastric banding, sleeve gastrectomy) or by causing malabsorption (Roux-en-Y gastric bypass, and duodenal switch with biliopancreatic diversion). No one surgery has been deemed more effective over others in terms of fertility outcomes. Bariatric surgery helps in improving all parameters of PCOS and metabolic syndrome greatly reducing the risk for cardiovascular events. A wait of 12-24 months before conceiving is advised so patient can achieve her weight-loss goals. A thorough evaluation and correction of micronutrient deficiencies before planning pregnancy is advised. Intrauterine growth restriction (IUGR), unexplained neonatal deaths have been seen with pregnancies conceived within a year of surgery. As per a 2016 systematic review, maternal pregnancy outcomes in postsurgery patients were better in terms of incidence of gestational diabetes and large for date infants vis-a-vis obese controls.

Management of Menstrual Disorders

Oligomenorrhea or secondary amenorrhea is not a worrisome symptom and does not require treatment unless the patient insists on it. A progesterone withdrawal bleeding can be induced with medroxyprogesterone acetate given in doses of 10 mg once daily for 7-10 days every month. In women with heavy prolonged bleeding, hirsutism, or women fearing pregnancy from the odd ovulation, combined oral contraceptives become the drug of choice. It also provides protection from endometrial hyperplasia. Benefits with oral contraceptive pills (OCPs) outweigh the risks posed by its use in PCOS women (level B evidence). However, relative contraindications for OCP use may exist at a higher frequency in such women. Long-term OCP use neither changes nor improves cardiometabolic risk. In the absence of other risk factors, women with PCOS are *not* at increased risk with OCPs (level C).

No differences are seen in the effectiveness or risk profiles among the various progestogens and when used in combination with a 20 μg versus a 30 μg daily dose of estrogen (level B). Subsequent fertility is not negatively affected by OCPs (level C).

Management of Hirsutism

Around 70% of women with PCOS are hirsute and adolescents and young adults are more likely to seek treatment for it. After ruling out other causes for hirsutism that require specific therapy, hirsutism due to PCOS can be treated either with pharmacotherapy or with ablative therapy. The most effective strategy is to combine systemic pharmacotherapy, which has a slow onset of effectiveness, with mechanical depilation (shaving, plucking, waxing, depilatory creams) or light-based (laser or pulsed-light) hair removal, which have instantaneous results.

Pharmacotherapy involves the use of oral contraceptive pills with or without antiandrogen agents. Oral contraceptive agents act in a three-pronged way by reducing androgen production (lower pituitary production of gonadotropins, thereby lowering LH induced ovarian androgen production), reducing androgen availability (increase hepatic SHBG production which binds excess free androgens) and reducing androgen action (direct receptor antagonist). There is no definitive evidence that the type of OCP determines efficacy of hirsutism control (level C). Prolonged (>6 months) medical therapy for hirsutism is necessary to document effectiveness (Level B). Antiandrogens (spironolactone, flutamide and finasteride) are added when after 6 months of OCP use, no significant improvement is seen in hirsutism scores. Flutamide is of limited value because of its dose-dependent hepatotoxicity (level B). Antiandrogens should not be used without effective contraception for risk of feminizing a male fetus (level B).

Shaving, plucking, waxing, depilatory creams are temporary ways of hair reduction with side effects like folliculitis, irritation, scarring, etc. Electrolysis is one of the most effective and permanent methods of hair removal, and may be an adjunct to hormonal treatment. However, electrolysis is now supplanted by use of laser techniques. The need for rapid methods of hair removal has led to the development of laser therapy for hirsutism. Several different lasers exist, including ruby, alexandrite, pulsed diode, and Q-switched yttrium-aluminum-garnet (YAG) lasers. Pulsed diode lasers are generally less expensive and more reliable than other laser sources for hair removal. Q-switched YAG lasers work well in patients with darker skin; however, these lasers are ineffective for long-term hair removal. Most patients experience a two- to six-month growth delay after a single treatment, and some have permanent hair removal after multiple treatments. Laser therapy works best on dark hair.

Management of Infertility

Infertility is one of the primary complaints in women with PCOS. Oligo-ovulation remains the chief cause for subfertility. As per the ESHRE-ASRM consensus meet in 2007, infertility treatment is four tiered. The first advice to all infertile PCOS women remains lifestyle modifications with the purpose of losing weight (as detailed above). Ovulation induction with oral agents and/or injectables is advised next. This is coupled with either timed intercourse or intrauterine insemination. Laparoscopic ovarian drilling forms the third line of management. *In vitro fertilization* (IVF) remains the final frontier of management.

Ovulation Induction

The following three points should be borne in mind when inducing ovulation in a woman with PCOS.
1. Before stimulating it is important to diagnosis and correctly categorize the type of anovulation since each will have an approach different from each other:
    - *Anovulatory group I*: Hypogonadotropic hypogonadism
    - *Anovulatory group II*: Normogonadotropic normogonadism
    - *Anovulatory group III*: Hypergonadotropic hypogonadism
    - Polycystic ovarian syndrome falls in group II anovulation and only in this group can the oral ovulation induction agents be used since oral agents require an intact pituitary acting on an active ovary.

2. The aim of ovulation induction in anovulatory or oligoovulatory PCOS is to achieve unifollicular ovulation. This is usually tricky as the FSH threshold required for unifollicular development is only slightly lower than multifollicular development leaving a very narrow margin of safety to work in which is often crossed when due care is not taken to fine tune the stimulation. This renders the PCOS woman vulnerable to the risks of ovarian hyperstimulation syndrome and multiple pregnancies.
3. Drugs commonly used for ovulation induction in PCOS are:
    - Clomiphene citrate (CC)
    - Letrozole
    - Tamoxifen
    - Clomiphene citrate + gonadotropins (Gn)
    - Gonadotropins.

Clomiphene citrate (CC): Clomiphene citrate is a nonsteroidal analogue of estradiol that exerts a positive influence on ovarian folliculogenesis by its estrogen receptor antagonistic activity so that the estrogen molecule ceases to act temporarily on the hypothalamus. By preventing negative feedback inhibition by estrogen on the hypothalamic receptors, it allows GnRH to be released in waves of greater amplitudes and frequency, which favors FSH release. These rising FSH levels initiate folliculogenesis.

Clomiphene citrate is a stereoisomer between two compounds, 38% of cis and 62% of trans-isomers. While the cis-isomer is a complete estrogen receptor antagonist, the trans-isomer has partial agonistic activity. The cis is a short-lived isomer with a half-life less than 24 hours and trans is longer lived lasting in the body for as long as 7 days after the last dose has been administered. The ovulation induction action of CC is due to its cis-isomer.

The starting dose of CC is 50 mg once daily started between day 2 and day 5 of the menstrual cycle given for 5 days. Ovulation occurs approximately 7 days after the last dose. Follicular monitoring with ultrasound can begin 5 days after the last dose. The monitoring should continue till about 2 weeks after the last dose to look for a delayed response. Ultrasonic evidence of ovulation could be—development of dominant follicle more than or equal to 17 mm followed by disappearance, reduction in size of dominant follicle by more than 5 mm, a change in the shape and appearance of internal echoes within the follicle, appearance of free fluid in the pouch of Douglas.

Response could also be monitored with serum progesterone levels 6–7 days after supposed ovulation. Values more than 3 ng/mL confirm ovulation.

Trouble shooting with clomiphene citrate: If the 50 mg dose fails to produce the desired result, the dose should be stepped up by another 50 mg and the cycle monitored till at least two weeks after the last dose. The highest FDA permissible dose that can be administered in a cycle is 750 mg. This means that the daily dose cannot be increased beyond 150 mg given for not more

than five days. If the woman fails to ovulate with the maximum permissible dose, a case of CC resistance is diagnosed. In such a situation, before jumping to the next step, ensure that the diagnosis of type II anovulation was correct. Thereafter undertake the following measures:
- Lifestyle modifications need to be stepped up.
- Metformin could be added to aid in correcting insulin resistance.
- Laparoscopic ovarian drilling may be advised in specific women with PCOS.
- Add gonadotropins.

If despite six cycles of successful ovulation after clomiphene, the woman fails to conceive, it is diagnosed as a case of *clomiphene failure*. Such cases are treated as any other case of unexplained infertility. After assessing semen, fallopian tubes and the uterine cavity, intrauterine insemination (IUI) is offered along with ovarian stimulation, preferably with gonadotropins.

Thin endometrium is likely, due to estrogen receptor blockade and is seen more often with higher doses of clomiphene. Hence, exogenous estradiol supplementation will not help. Receptor blockade generally clears by day 4-5 of last dose. Endometrium usually bounces back to normal by the day of ovulation. If it persists, rule out other causes of thin endometrium like endometritis, synechiae, etc. Lower doses of clomiphene coupled with Gn, tamoxifen, letrozole or all gonadotropin cycle can help in alleviating clomiphene's antiestrogenic effect on the endometrium.

Cysts with clomiphene citrate are mostly seen in women with regularly ovulating women with short cycles, advanced age or poor ovarian reserve. Sometimes also with use of higher doses of CC or in late start cycles. Corrective measures include administering clomiphene citrate in the minimum effective dose in women with oligoovulatory infertility and not in women with unexplained infertility with poor reserves. In the latter, starting CC later than day 3 or with 100 mg dose should be avoided.

Letrozole: Letrozole is an aromatase inhibitor that prevents the conversion of androgens to estrogens. By lowering estrogen levels, it maintains FSH levels above the threshold required for folliculogenesis for longer intervals than normal allowing the development of one or more follicles. It is given in doses of 2.5-7.5 mg for 5 days in the early follicular phase. Endometrial thinning is seen with higher doses but owing to its short half-life, is quickly reversed upon stopping the drug. It has been seen as an effective alternative to clomiphene citrate in PCOS women.

Tamoxifen: It is a selective estrogen receptor antagonist that has a mechanism of action similar to clomiphene citrate? It exerts a partial estrogenic effect on endometrial estrogen receptors, hence endometrial thinning is not seen with its use. It is used in daily doses of 40-80 mg for 5 days given in the early follicular phase. Larger prospective comparative studies needed to recommend tamoxifen over CC.

Gonadotropins: They are considered second line ovulation induction agents in PCOS. The indications for its use are CC failure, CC resistance, persistence of thin endometrium and repeated cyst formation with CC. Usually a chronic low dose step-up protocol is helpful in these women. The starting dose is determined by BMI, with thinner women requiring lower doses than obese women. A typical starting dose would be 50-75 IU in women with BMIs between 20 kg/m² and 24 kg/m². In more obese women, a starting dose of 125-150 IU might be more appropriate. The chosen starting dose is given daily for 6-7 days after which response is monitored through a transvaginal scan. Gonadotropin dose is lowered if the follicular response is excessive and continued in similar doses for a couple of days if one to two follicles have gained dominance. If no follicular response is seen despite 7 days of initial dose, the same dose is continued for another 5-7 days. It is important to withhold the urge to step-up the dose at this stage since the safety margin between the development of a couple of follicles and multiple follicles is very narrow. Experts' advice on raising the dose of gonadotropins by increments of not more than 50% of baseline after at least ten days of the same dose has produced no response. No one kind of gonadotropin [urinary or recombinant, FSH or human menopausal gonadotropin (hMG)] is preferred, since they are considered equivalent in terms of effectiveness or their adverse effect profile. The gonadotropins that are available in a pen form, allow for dose increments of as small as 12.5 units and offer a distinct advantage in fine tuning stimulation in PCOS women.

Laparoscopic ovarian drilling (LOD): The indication for ovarian drilling in a case of PCOS is very specific and that is clomiphene resistance. LOD is preferred over gonadotropins in women with CC resistance when other indications for laparoscopic evaluation are present like adnexal masses, uterine lesions, tubal pathology, etc. It is also a good choice in women who live in a different city and cannot manage the frequent visits required in monitoring a gonadotropin cycle. The other advantages of LOD over gonadotropins are the complete avoidance of multiple pregnancies, ovarian hyperstimulation syndrome (OHSS) and follicular and hormonal monitoring and the possibility of multiple natural pregnancy trials that it affords. LOD is done in the operation theater (OT) setting with a monopolar needle electrode that punctures the ovarian stroma at four to six sites and delivers 40 W of current at a depth of 4 mm for 4 seconds to ablate the stromal tissue. This reduces intraovarian androgens, which act locally to improve follicular estrogen-androgen ratio and at the pituitary level to improve FSH-LH ratio. Both these effects are expected to bring about folliculogenesis. Spontaneous ovulation is seen in about 50-60% of correctly chosen women. It is most successful in thin women with high LH. It is less successful in women with BMI more than 30 kg/m², high testosterone levels and in women with duration of infertility more than 3 years.

Intrauterine insemination or in vitro fertilization in polycystic ovarian syndrome: If after six ovulatory cycles and timed intercourse, no conception has occurred resort to intrauterine insemination, provided the rest of infertility work-up in the couple is normal. IVF is indicated when 4 IUIs coupled with induced ovulation have failed.

Role of Other Medicines

Metformin:
- Insulin sensitizer that does not cause hypoglycemia. It has gastrointestinal side effects.
- Dose is 850 mg twice a day.
- Given in PCOS women with abnormal glucose tolerance test (GTT), women who fail to show weight reduction with lifestyle modifications or in women showing clomiphene resistance. Is more effective in inducing ovulation when given in thin PCOS women along with clomiphene citrate. Also given to women at risk for OHSS undergoing stimulation for IVF.
- Glucose intolerant PCOS women who get pregnant should continue metformin to avoid gestational diabetes mellitus.

Dopamine agonists (DA): Dopamine agonists like bromocriptine and cabgolin were used in the past to overcome clomiphene resistance. But later evidence did not show any improvements in ovulation rates with use of DAs in PCOS women with normoprolactinemia. ASRM-ESHRE consensus meets have not endorsed the use of dopamine agonists in PCOS women with normoprolactinemia for clomiphene resistance.

However, in prevention of ovarian hyperstimulation syndrome, numerous studies have found dopamine agonists very effective, although have not so in treating it. No conclusions can be made regarding the most effective DA, the optimal dose or the most appropriate drug regimen for preventing OHSS.

Myo or chiro-inositol: Inositols function as second messenger systems for insulin action. They lower insulin levels in blood by increasing cellular sensitivity to insulin. Two inositol isomers, myo-inositol (MI) and D-chiro-inositol (DCI) have been proven to be effective in PCOS treatment, by improving insulin resistance, serum androgen levels and many features of the metabolic syndrome. The combination of MI or DCI in the ratio of 40:1 has been available for the past few years commercially. It is used as a once daily tablet for up to 6 months. Whether or not the improvement in biochemical parameters translate into an improvement in live births, remains to be seen by further randomized controlled studies.

CONCLUSION
- Polycystic ovary syndrome is a clinically heterogeneous condition having a multifactorial etiology.

- It is best defined as a condition of androgen excess that causes either ovulatory disturbance and/or polycystic ovarian morphology.
- It manifests clinically in different ways through different age groups.
- Management rests largely on lifestyle modification.
- Pharmacotherapy and surgery is reserved for special situations.
- Oral contraceptives are used for menstrual cycle regulation, hirsutism and for contraception in PCOS women. Although relative contraindications for its use are more likely to exist in PCOS women, they are largely considered safe for use.
- Infertility management consists of correctly categorizing the anovulatory disorder and then taking measures for inducing ovulation.
- The first line in infertility management remains lifestyle modification.
- Pharmacotherapy is instituted after lifestyle modifications have been instituted.
- Clomiphene citrate is the first line oral agent for infertility management. Letrozole and tamoxifen are equally effective. Gonadotropins form the second line of drugs to be used in ovulation induction in PCOS women.
- Laparoscopic ovarian drilling is advised in cases of clomiphene citrate resistance.
- Intrauterine insemination is coupled with ovarian stimulation in cases of clomiphene failure after confirming normalcy of semen and fallopian tubes.
- *In vitro* fertilization is reserved for PCOS women who have failed to conceive despite four cycles of IUI.

SUGGESTED READING

1. Amer SA, Li TC, Ledger WL. Ovulation induction using laparoscopic ovarian drilling in women with polycystic ovarian syndrome: predictors of success. Hum Reprod. 2004;19(8):1719-24.
2. Armstrong C. ACOG Guidelines on Pregnancy after Bariatric Surgery. Am Fam Physician. 2010;81(7):905-6.
3. Baumgarten M, Polanski L, Campbell B, et al. Do dopamine agonists prevent or reduce the severity of ovarian hyperstimulation syndrome in women undergoing assisted reproduction? A systematic review and meta-analysis. Hum Fertil (Camb). 2013;16(3):168-74.
4. Franks S. When should an insulin sensitizing agent be used in the treatment of polycystic ovary syndrome? Clin Endocrinol (Oxf). 2011;74(2):148-51.
5. Morley LC, Tang T, Yasmin E, et al. Insulin-sensitizing drugs (metformin, rosiglitazone, pioglitazone, D-chiro-inositol) for women with polycystic ovary syndrome, oligo amenorrhea and subfertility. Cochrane Database Syst Rev. 2017;11:CD003053.
6. Rueda-Clausen CF, Padwal RS. Pharmacotherapy for weight loss. BMJ. 2014;348:g3526.
7. Satwik R. Adolescent Acne and Hirsutism. In: Ganguli I, Khullar H (Eds). Obstetrics and Gynecology. Case based approach. Kolkata: TreeLife Media; 2015.
8. Skubleny D, Switzer NJ, Gill RS, et al. The Impact of bariatric surgery on polycystic ovary syndrome: a systematic review and meta-analysis. Obes Surg. 2016;26(1):169-76.

9. The Amsterdam ESHRE/ASRM-Sponsored 3rd PCOS Consensus Workshop Group. Consensus on women's health aspects of polycystic ovary syndrome (PCOS). Hum Reprod. 2012;27(1):14-24.
10. The Rotterdam ESHRE/ASRM sponsored PCOS consensus workshop group. Revised 2003 consensus on diagnostic criteria and long-term health risks related to polycystic ovary syndrome (PCOS). Hum Reprod. 2004;19(1):41-7.
11. Thessaloniki ESHRE/ASRM-Sponsored PCOS Consensus Workshop Group1. Consensus on infertility treatment related to polycystic ovary syndrome. Hum Reprod. 2008;23(3):462-77.

CHAPTER 12

Management of an Infertile Couple

Abha Majumdar, Neeti Tiwari

INTRODUCTION

Infertility is defined as inability to conceive after 1 year of regular unprotected intercourse. In some conditions though an earlier evaluation is warranted, e.g. age of female partner more than 35 years, history of irregular cycles, known case of endometriosis, or history of pelvic surgery. Similarly in males, if the semen analysis is already known to be abnormal on two or more occasions one does not need to wait for 1 year to start treatment.

It is imperative to evaluate the couple and not target a single partner alone at a time; hence, evaluation of both the partners should start simultaneously. Being infertile often has a social stigma associated with it, especially for the female partner and sometimes might also interfere with a couples privacy or emotional life, causing a lot of stress between the couple. Therefore, it is pertinent for the treating clinician to provide psychological and emotional support throughout the process of evaluation and management of such couples.

EVALUATION OF FEMALE PARTNER

In women, the causes of infertility include ovulatory disorders (30%), tubal and pelvic pathology (40%), uncommon causes like uterine cavity abnormalities (5-10%), and yet in another 20% no cause is found and is categorized as unexplained infertility.

Clinical History

A detailed history taking and examination can identify the cause of infertility and hence investigation can be done in a focused way. In female, relevant history includes the following:
- Duration of infertility and results of any prior investigations.
- Sexual history—coital frequency, any sexual dysfunction as well as the knowledge of fertile period. Use of vaginal lubricants or vaginal douches immediately after intercourse.

- Menstrual history—age at menarche, cycle characteristics, significant dysmenorrhea along with history of primary or secondary amenorrhea.
- Obstetric history—previous pregnancies, if any and their outcomes and complications.
- Contraceptive history
- Past medical and surgical history—history of prolonged illness or previous surgery or hospitalization. Any medical illness, e.g. diabetes mellitus, hypertension. Specifically one must ask for history of pelvic inflammatory diseases, sexually transmitted diseases, and tuberculosis.
- History of thyroid disorders, galactorrhea and hirsutism, or history of excessive weight gain or loss.
- Occupational exposure to known environmental hazards.
- History of any addictions such as nicotine, alcohol, and drugs.
- Family history of consanguinity, congenital abnormalities, mental retardation, early menopause, or reproductive failure.

Physical Examination

A detailed general physical examination should be followed by pelvic examination at the first visit.

- *General examination*: Height, weight, and body mass index (BMI), secondary sexual characteristics, breast examination for development, or galactorrhea. Look for abnormal or excessive hair growth over face, chest, and abdomen. Thyroid gland should be specifically examined.
- *Systemic examination*: Lungs and heart to be examined.
- *Abdominal examination*: Organomegaly and surgical scars need to be noted.
- *Pelvic examination*: Vaginal introitus, size, and shape of clitoris, hymen. Presence of vaginal discharge on per speculum examination to be noted. On per vaginum examination, look for direction, size, shape, and mobility of uterus, forniceal tenderness, or adnexal mass.

Investigations

The aim of investigations is to identify the cause of infertility, which can then be targeted. In female partner, we look for ovulatory function, tubal patency, and rule out any uterine pathology. Routine preconceptional tests should also be included in the initial evaluation.

General Investigations

The investigations include blood group and Rh typing, hemogram, thalassemia screen, blood sugar fasting or random, thyroid profile, and rubella serology. Infectious screen includes evaluation of human immunodeficiency virus (HIV)-I and -II, hepatitis B and C, and Venereal Disease Research

Laboratory (VDRL) status in husband and wife. These investigations are important when assisted reproductive procedures are to be undertaken where gamete handling needs to be done.

When to suspect an ovulatory problem?

Regular menstrual cycles of 24–35 days are consistent with ovulation in 97% of cases. If a patient presents with oligomenorrhea or amenorrhea, she is either having oligoovulation or anovulation and no test are required to prove it. Most common cause of oligomenorrhea is polycystic ovarian syndrome (PCOS). Other common causes are hyperprolactinemia, hypothyroidism, and premature ovarian failure. Secondary amenorrhea, i.e. complete absence of menses for 6 months or more can be due to hypogonadotropic hypogonadism, premature ovarian failure, PCOS, and severe hyperprolactinemia.

When to confirm ovulation?

Although regular menses strongly suggest ovulatory cycles investigations for ovulatory function is definitely warranted in infertile women.

- *Midluteal serum progesterone measurement*: A single blood test used most commonly to confirm ovulation is the estimation of serum progesterone (P4). Serum concentration of P4 more than 3 ng/mL is usually taken as presumptive evidence of recent ovulation. It should be measured a week before the expected menses or around day 21 or 22 in a woman with regular cycles.
- *Urinary luteinizing hormone (LH) kits* can be used by the woman herself to identify midcycle LH surge in urine and hence predict impending ovulation, which should occur within 2 days of the test being positive. It identifies the fertile period in a woman's cycles without the need for her to go to a laboratory for testing. However, repetitive use of LH kits can be expensive.
- *Follicular monitoring by transvaginal ultrasound*: Follicular monitoring is generally used during ovulation induction or ovarian stimulation of women who do not appear to ovulate regularly or where we plan to assist conception by adding intrauterine insemination (IUI) or in vitro fertilization (IVF). This method detects ovulation most precisely. Progressive increase in follicular size with development of triple-layered endometrium followed by sudden disappearance of follicle, appearance of fluid in cul-de-sac, and homogenization of endometrium gives a presumptive diagnosis of ovulation.
- *Endometrial biopsy*: Secretory endometrium on histopathology of endometrial biopsy is suggestive of action of progesterone in luteal phase and hence retrospectively proves ovulation. The test being invasive is not used for documentation of ovulation anymore. In infertile women, endometrial biopsy is taken only when some pathology like endometrial hyperplasia or chronic endometritis are suspected or one wants to rule out luteal phase defect as the cause of infertility.

- *Basal body temperature (BBT) measurement*: It was used to document ovulation for diagnostic purpose as well as to time intercourse. In cycles monitored with BBT period of highest fertility spans 7 days prior to rise in BBT. Biphasic pattern on BBT is associated with ovulatory cycles and anovulatory cycles have monophasic pattern but often ovulatory women also record monophasic or interpretable pattern. Maintaining BBT is often difficult, tedious, and may cause a lot of stress, hence is no longer recommended for evaluation of ovulatory function.

Tubal Evaluation

Since tubal evaluation is an invasive test, semen analysis of male partner should be done beforehand. In case of severe oligoasthenoteratozoospermia (OATs) or azoospermia with presence of testicular or epididymal sperm, couples can have their own genetic child by the process of IVF. For such couples, tubal evaluation is not required. However, if such couples need the use of donor sperm then tubal patency should be confirmed before donor insemination. The different ways to assess tubal patency are hysterosalpingography (HSG), hysterosalpingo-contrast-sonography (HyCoSy), and laparoscopy with chromopertubation.

Hysterosalpingography

Hysterosalpingography using water-soluble media is the standard first-line investigation for tubal evaluation. The uterine cavity is delineated in initial images while later images outline the tubes and show peritoneal spill. HSG is usually planned between day 6 and 11 of cycle to ensure absence of pregnancy and facilitate better visualization of uterine cavity. Active pelvic infection, pregnancy, and any known allergies to the contrast medium should be ruled out. The proximal tubal block on HSG is often due to cornual spasm; hence, HSG is more specific for diagnosing distal or midtubal as compared to proximal occlusion. Postprocedure antibiotic prophylaxis, e.g. doxycycline is recommended.

Hysterosalpingo-contrast-sonography

The HyCoSy is pelvic ultrasonography combined with uterine instillation of saline or contrast media. Presence of fluid in cul-de-sac confirms tubal patency, but it does not differentiate between unilateral and bilateral patency. Simultaneous sonographic visualization of uterus, uterine cavity, and adnexal structures along with tubal patency are an advantage of HyCoSy.

Who needs laparoscopy in infertility workup?

Laparoscopy with chromopertubation has been considered as the "gold standard" for tubal evaluation hence whenever there is a problem detected on HSG, final confirmation and further treatment are done on laparoscopy. Besides these, other indications of laparoscopy are as follows:

- Suspected pelvic problems diagnosed on ultrasound as presence of a cyst, mass, or pelvic adhesions
- Suspected congenital malformations of the genital tract
- Previous surgery on abdomen or pelvis (laparoscopic or open surgery)
- Duration of infertility of more than 4–5 years
- Despite having all factors normal and patent tubes on HSG, the couple fails to conceive for over 1 year of active management of infertility.

Evaluation of Uterus

A simple *two-dimensional transvaginal ultrasound* should be done at the beginning of treatment to rule out submucosal fibroids, intrauterine adhesions, endometrial polyps, septum, etc. *Three-dimensional (3D) ultrasound* provides a better visualization of uterine cavity and hence is good when Müllerian anomalies or intracavitary lesions are suspected. *Saline hysterosonography (SHS)* is ultrasound combined with saline infusion of uterine cavity, it improves the delineation of cavity and hence is more efficient in diagnosing submucosal fibroids and polyps. 3D SHS is comparable to hysteroscopy in diagnosing intrauterine adhesions. The gold standard for evaluation of uterine cavity is *hysteroscopy* and is recommended for diagnosis as well as treatment for a suspected intrauterine pathology.

Other Investigations for Female Partner

Who should be tested for ovarian reserve?

Ovarian reserve needs to be tested in the following conditions:
- Age more than 35 years
- Family history of early menopause
- History of surgery done on one or both ovaries or removal of one ovary, chemotherapy, or pelvic irradiation
- Poor response to ovarian stimulation in past
- Unexplained infertility
- Those undergoing treatment with assisted reproductive technology (ART).

The tests done to assess ovarian reserve in common practice are day 2/3 serum follicle stimulating hormone (FSH) and estradiol (E2), along with antral follicle count (AFC) with ovarian volume and serum anti-Müllerian hormone (AMH). AFC and AMH can be done generally on any day of the menstrual cycle.
- *Day 2/3 FSH and estradiol*: Serum measurements of FSH and estradiol are done in early follicular phase commonly to assess ovarian reserve. A higher FSH level predicts a poor ovarian reserve (upper limit 10–25 IU/mL). High level of basal serum estradiol (>80 pg/mL) along with normal FSH is also associated with poor ovarian response.

- *Antral follicle count*: AFC is preferably done on cycle day 2–8 by transvaginal route and serves as a direct ovarian reserve marker. However, it can be done on any day of the cycle, if needed, and abdominal ultrasound can be used in special circumstances. A low AFC (range 3–10) has been associated with poor ovarian response to stimulation.
- *Serum AMH*: AMH, secreted by granulosa cells of growing follicles, is another direct measure of the ovarian reserve. AMH can be measured on any day of cycle as cyclic variation is minimal. Low AMH level predicts poor ovarian response to stimulation while high AMH level predicts hyperresponse.

Other Hormonal Evaluations

Some hormonal evaluations are required in specific conditions:
- *Prolactin*: Repeated high-serum prolactin levels in presence of delayed cycles and absence of polycystic ovaries indicate the possibility of pathological hyperprolactinemia causing anovulation. In these cases, there is lack of rise in progesterone levels in second half of menstrual cycles. Careful drug intake history especially those for mental or psychological illnesses need to be taken to rule out iatrogenic hyperprolactinemia.
- *Thyroid profile*: Though thyroid profile is included in routine prenatal screening in our population, it should not be missed in women with irregular cycles or where thyroid disorder is suspected.
- *Serum androgen measurement*: Circulating androgens (free and total testosterone and dehydroepiandrosterone sulfate, i.e. DHEAS), SHBG, and 17-hydroxyprogesterone are measured in case of severe hirsutism or acne. 17-hydroxyprogesterone is usually elevated in late-onset congenital adrenal hyperplasia (CAH) because of 21-hydroxylase deficiency. High levels of DHEAS suggest pathological conditions involving the adrenal gland.

Postcoital Test

Postcoital test (PCT) is done for evaluation of cervical factor and indirectly the male factor in an ovulating patient. It is best to perform the test around the time of ovulation and 8–12 hours after the coitus. The cervical mucus is collected from the cervical canal with an artery forceps, placed on a slide, and examination is done under high-power (40×) microscope. At least one motile sperm per high-power field constitute a positive test. Negative PCT is seen with severe astheno- or oligospermia or low-semen volume. No sperm seen on repeated PCT despite a normal semen analysis is suggestive of coital problem. Improper timing or very thick cervical mucus can also lead to immotile sperms. This test is subjective with poor-predictive value hence hardly changes management. PCT is no longer routinely recommended in infertility workup.

Genetic Assessment

In women with primary or secondary amenorrhea with ovarian failure, karyotype is done to rule out Turner's syndrome. Fragile X syndrome should also be excluded in patients with premature ovarian failure with test for FMR gene mutation.

EVALUATION OF MALE PARTNER

Male factor is responsible for 30-40% of infertility in couples. In 20% of infertile couples, male factor is solely responsible for infertility; whereas in another 10-20%, it is present with female factor infertility.

Clinical History

At the first visit itself, a detailed history should be taken from male partner.
- Duration of infertility and prior fertility.
- *Sexual history*: Coital frequency and timing, any associated problems, e.g. erectile dysfunction or loss of libido.
- *Developmental history*: Any congenital malformation of genitalia, cryptorchidism, and delayed onset of puberty.
- *Medical history*: History of mumps orchitis, sexually transmitted diseases. History of medical conditions like diabetes, upper respiratory diseases, or any prolonged illnesses.
- *Surgical history*: History of herniorrhaphy particularly in childhood. Any history of genitourinary surgeries, instrumentation, or trauma.
- *Addiction*: History of smoking, alcohol intake, and use of recreational drugs or anabolic steroids.
- Occupational or environmental exposure to toxins such as heat and chemicals, which can disrupt endocrine system.
- *Family history*: Infertility in other male members of the family, history of consanguinity.

Physical Examination

Male partner is examined only if semen analysis is abnormal.

General Examination

Vitals such as pulse rate, blood pressure along with height, weight, and BMI, secondary sexual characteristics including body habitus, hair distribution, breast, and thyroid gland examination should be undertaken.

Genital Examination

Shape and size of penis, prepuce and position of external urethral meatus should be seen. One must palpate for presence of vas deferens, epididymis, and volume of testis, which can be assessed either by the help of ultrasound or by Prader's orchidometer (normal volume 20–25 mL). Looking for varicocele and hydrocele is also essential. A varicocele, which is not seen clinically but only diagnosed by ultrasound usually, requires no treatment.

Investigations

Semen analysis is the first investigation required in male partner and other tests are required only, if initial semen analysis report is abnormal.

Semen Analysis

Semen sample is collected in the laboratory by masturbation after 2–7 days of abstinence. It can also be collected at home or during intercourse in a condom without spermicidal and should reach laboratory within 1 hour of collection. Semen analysis includes parameters like volume, pH, sperm concentration, vitality, motility, and morphology the normal values of which according to World Health Organization (WHO) manual 2010 are given in Table 12.1.

- *Volume*: Low-semen volume can be due to faulty collection, retrograde ejaculation, or absence or blockage of the seminal vesicles or ejaculatory duct in the prostrate or congenital bilateral absence of vas deferens (CBAVD). Active inflammation of accessory glands can lead to high volume.
- *pH*: Lower pH with low volume and azoospermia is due to ejaculatory duct obstruction or CBAVD.
- *Sperm concentration*: Sperm concentration less than 5 million/mL is known as severe oligozoospermia, whereas azoospermia is complete absence of spermatozoa in the ejaculate. To rule out interobserver and intraobserver variations, semen analysis should be repeated after a month if found abnormal. In case of azoospermia, the semen sample should be centrifuged and pellet examined to rule out complete absence

Table 12.1: Reference values of semen analysis according to World Health Organization (WHO) manual 2010.

Criteria	Reference value
Volume	≥1.5 mL
Total sperm number	≥39 millions/ejaculate
Sperm concentration	≥15 millions/mL
Total motility	≥40%
Progressive motility	≥32%
Normal morphology	≥4%
Vitality	≥58%

of sperms or confirm the presence of few sperms in the pellet known as cryptozoospermia.
- *Sperm motility*: Motility is graded as (a) progressive where spermatozoa are moving actively in forward direction, (b) nonprogressive where spermatozoa are motile but without progression, and (c) immotile. It is only the progressively motile fraction of sperm, which cause natural conception.
- *Sperm vitality*: It is an important parameter when sperm motility is low or all the sperms are immotile.
- *Sperm morphology*: Head, neck, midpiece, and tail are examined in detail for morphology and classified as normal or abnormal according to Kruger's strict criteria (Tygerberg). According to these criteria even if 5% of sperm have normal morphology, the sperm has normal fertilizing ability. Abnormal sperm have lower fertilization potential and may be associated with Deoxyribo-nucleic acid (DNA) defects.
- *Seminal fructose*: Absence of fructose in semen suggests either seminal vesicle agenesis/dysfunction or ejaculatory duct obstruction as fructose is secreted by seminal vesicles.
- *Pyospermia/leukocytospermia or presence of "round cells" in semen*: Both leukocytes (pus cells) and immature spermatozoa appear as round cells under wet mount. It is very important to distinguish between the two because presence of leukocytes in semen indicates infection or inflammation. According to WHO, pyospermia, which is also referred to as leukocytospermia, is defined as concentration of round cells more than 1 million/mL. In such cases, pus cells should be differentiated from immature sperms presenting as round cells, by the use of peroxidase stain.

Other Investigations for Infertile Male Partner

These investigations are recommended only if initial semen analysis shows abnormal findings.

Scrotal Ultrasound

It is generally indicated where clinical examination is ambiguous, e.g. doubtful testicular mass, high up testis, or small scrotal sac. It should also be done in patients at risk of testicular cancer, e.g. cryptorchidism or history of tumor in one testis. Transrectal ultrasound (TRUS) is usually done to assess prostate or ejaculatory ducts.

Hormonal Analysis

In men with severe oligospermia or azoospermia, serum FSH and total serum testosterone are tested. Low-serum levels of FSH with low testosterone are associated with hypogonadotropic hypogonadism, whereas high levels of FSH and LH with low or normal testosterone indicate hypergonadotropic hypogonadism or testicular failure.

Postejaculation Urine Analysis

Retrograde ejaculation needs to be ruled out in patients who repeatedly have very low semen volume. The postejaculation urine is collected and centrifuged at 300 g for 10 minutes. The pellet is examined for sperms at 400× magnification and presence of even one sperm in patients with azoospermia confirm the diagnosis of retrograde ejaculation.

Sperm DNA Fragmentation Tests

The DNA fragmentation refers to damaged or denatured sperm DNA during spermatogenesis or during its transport. There are direct or indirect methods to test sperm DNA fragmentation.
- Direct tests are *single cell gel electrophoresis assay (COMET)* and *terminal deoxynucleotidyl transferase dUTP (Deoxyuridine triphosphate) nick end labeling assay (TUNEL)*, which analyze number of breaks in DNA.
- *Sperm chromatin structure assay (SCSA)* is the indirect test, which identifies abnormal chromatin structure, as it has increased sensitivity to acid denaturation.

Though sperm DNA damage has been associated with poor reproductive outcome and recurrent spontaneous abortions, it is not routinely recommended due to limited clinical significance.

Genetic Testing

Karyotyping and Y-chromosome microdeletion are indicated in patients with severe OATs or azoospermia with testicular failure. Genetic counseling and preimplantation genetic diagnosis are recommended where one plans to use these sperm by the help of IVF. In patients with CBAVD, it is important to test for cystic fibrosis transmembrane receptor (CFTR) gene mutation as 85% of these infertile men carry one or two CFTR gene mutation. If positive then female partner is tested and in case she is found to be carrier of the same mutation, there is 25% chance of their child being affected with cystic fibrosis or CBAVD.

TREATMENT OF SPECIFIC DISORDERS

Disorders of Ovulation

Polycystic Ovarian Syndrome

This condition has been discussed in detail in Chapter 11. When women with PCOS present with anovulatory infertility, it is only then that they require help with ovulation induction. These women are quite commonly obese and if it is so, lifestyle modification with weight reduction may restore ovulation as well as fertility for this subset. However, weight reduction is not easy and it may not restore ovulation for all. In that case, the first-line drug for ovulation induction is clomiphene citrate (CC) in incremental doses in subsequent cycles till ovulation is achieved. The other oral ovulation induction agents used in common practice are either aromatase inhibitors such as letrozole or selective estrogen receptor modulator like CC such as tamoxifen. Gonadotropins are reserved for patients where either of the oral agents fails to induce ovulation or conception. Laparoscopic ovarian drilling of ovaries is also performed with the aim to reduce intraovarian androgen level in clomiphene-resistant cases, which helps to either induce spontaneous ovulation or makes these patients sensitive to clomiphene postdrilling.

Hyperprolactinemia

It can present with both oligomenorrhea and amenorrhea depending on severity of condition. Galactorrhea though pathognomonic of this condition is present in less than half the cases. Certain drugs like phenothiazines, butyrophenones, cimetidine can lead to hyperprolactinemia on prolonged intake hence one should not miss asking about them. In 40% of cases, hyperprolactinemia is associated with prolactin secreting benign tumors called prolactinomas, hence a computed tomography (CT) scan or magnetic resonance imaging (MRI) head should be ordered, if serum prolactin is more than 100 ng/dL. Dopamine receptor agonist such as bromocriptine or cabergoline is the most commonly used drugs for idiopathic hyperprolactinemia and microprolactinomas. Dopamine receptor agonist alone can restore ovulatory function and menstruation and hence is the first-line therapy for anovulatory infertility with hyperprolactinemia. Those who fail to achieve pregnancy on dopamine receptor agonist alone need gonadotropins.

Thyroid Disorders

Both hypothyroidism and hyperthyroidism can present with oligomenorrhea and amenorrhea with associated ovulatory disturbances leading to infertility. Hypothyroidism is treated with thyroxine replacement, which is continued during pregnancy also. Treatment of hyperthyroidism is with carbimazole, which is continued safely during pregnancy or can be replaced with propylthiouracil, which has long enjoyed the reputation of being safer in pregnancy.

Endometriosis

Blood supply to the affected ovary can be altered in endometriosis leading to oligoovulation and anovulation. Endometriosis is also associated with luteinized unruptured follicle syndrome, early demise of the corpus luteum (luteolysis) and oocyte maturation defects, which further hamper the chances of conception. When a patient with endometriosis comes with infertility role of medical management is limited. Laparoscopy is not only required for endometriotic cystectomy or fulguration of endometriotic implants, but also gives an opportunity for adhesiolysis and pelvic reconstruction to improve chances of spontaneous pregnancy as tubo-ovarian relationship is often altered due to adhesions. After laparoscopy depending on the stage of disease, tubal status, and ovarian reserve, further management is planned. Patients can be left to try naturally for 3-6 months or taken up for ovarian stimulation and IUI or sent for IVF in case of advanced disease with low-ovarian reserve. Gonadotropin-releasing hormone (GnRH) agonists like leuprolide or goserelin are most commonly used drugs for endometriosis. They lead to hypogonadotropic hypogonadic state, which leads to atrophy of the endometriotic implants. If given after laparoscopy, it takes away the opportunity for the couple to conceive when the chances are maximum, hence GnRH agonist depots should be given postsurgically only if there is significant residual disease left after surgery and one wants to proceed with IVF. Other medical agents like oral contraceptive pills, progestational drugs, danazol, and dienogest, which are used for pain relief and other symptoms in endometriosis find very limited use in infertility.

Hypogonadotropic Hypogonadism

These patients present with primary or secondary amenorrhea due to nonfunction of gonads secondary to deficiency of pituitary and hypothalamic stimulation. History of acute stress, illness, anorexia, weight loss, or severe exercise is important. Congenital form can be associated with anosmia also known as Kallmann syndrome. History of severe postpartum hemorrhage (PPH) preceding amenorrhea suggests Sheehan's syndrome. A CT scan or MRI brain should be ordered in these patients to rule out any space-occupying lesion. In hypogonadotropic hypogonadism, both FSH and LH are required to induce ovulation hence human menopausal gonadotropin (HMG), which is a combination of both gonadotropin is preferred for inducing ovulation.

Premature Ovarian Insufficiency or Failure

If an amenorrheic patient has low or normal endogenous estradiol levels with high FSH more than 40 mIU/mL on two occasions, the diagnosis of ovarian failure or premature ovarian failure (POF) is made. These patients need hormone replacement therapy in the form of cyclical estrogen and progestogen to get regular cycles till the age of natural menopause. Fertility is possible only by IVF with the help of donor oocytes. However, rising FSH levels with oligomenorrhoea cycles and low AMH indicate premature ovarian insufficiency (POI) and ovulation sometimes can be induced with the help of oral ovulation-inducing agents as well as gonadotropins in these women.

Treatment of Tubal Factor Infertility

Three modes of treatment are available:
- *Expectant management*: In cases where a unilateral tube is patent or both tubes are patent but convoluted and unhealthy, superovulation with IUI can be tried for few cycles hoping that the tubes may be able to transport a fertilized oocyte to the uterus.
- *Surgical approach*: Different procedures are recommended depending upon the level of block:
  - *Cornual block*: Bilateral cornual block on HSG is often due to cornual spasm and it is not uncommon to find these tubes patent on laparoscopy. However, if the block is confirmed during laparoscopy, hysteroscopic cannulation is the procedure of choice and almost 75–80% of the blocks can be negotiated successfully.
  - *Midsegment block*: End-to-end anastomosis can be tried but there could be multiple blocks, hence it works favorably only for tubal recanalization poststerilization. Pathological midtubal blocks have the worst prognosis even after surgical repair as these tubes have generally lost their structural as well as functional ability.
  - *Distal block and hydrosalpinx*: Laparoscopic fimbrial dilatation and fimbriolysis (removal of adhesions around the fimbria to make it free) are done for distal block. In case of hydrosalpinx, neosalpingostomy is tried where a new ostium is made to cover the entire surface of ovary to facilitate egg pickup. When the tube is grossly damaged in case of hydrosalpinx or pyosalpinx either clipping or removal of tube is advised to improve the chances of success in IVF.
  - *Peritubal or perifimbrial adhesions*: Fallopian tubes may be adherent to pelvic wall, ovaries, uterus, omentum, or even bowel due to endometriosis, postsurgical adhesions, or old infection. Laparoscopic adhesiolysis is done to restore tubo-ovarian relationship.
- *Assisted reproductive technology (ART)*: With the development of IVF, the role of tubal surgery has become limited. Whenever tubes are found to be irreparably damaged, IVF is now the preferred procedure of choice for successful fertility. In women with advanced age or poor ovarian reserve, one may bypass laparoscopy after tubal block seen on HSG and proceed for IVF directly.

Treatment of Male Factor Infertility

Lifestyle Changes

Sometimes certain lifestyle factors may be responsible for poor semen parameters. Counseling should be done to avoid smoking, alcohol abuse, recreational drugs, anabolic steroids, and excessive exercise. Weight loss is important in obese male.

Medical Management

This has a very limited role and is generally used in following conditions:
- *Hypogonadotropic hypogonadism*: These men generally present with azoospermia and have low or normal testosterone with very low FSH and LH. These men can be treated with gonadotropin replacement. The initial pituitary gonadotropin, which stimulates testicular function, is LH which acts on Leydig cells to stimulate production of testosterone. Human chorionic gonadotropin (hCG) simulates LH function and is long acting hence is used in place of LH in doses of 1,500–2,000 units thrice a week for 3-4 months till serum testosterone levels are seen to increase. At this stage in the presence of testosterone pituitary, FSH induces spermatogenesis by stimulating the Sertoli cells. Therefore to attain spermatogenesis either injection FSH (150 units alternate day) is used along with hCG or injection HMG (combination of FSH and LH) is given in doses of 75-150 units thrice a week for 6-12 months till sperm production starts and they begin to appear in semen. Depending on the sperm count, one can conceive naturally or may require assistance of IUI or IVF for conception.
- *Obese males with low testosterone to estradiol ratio*: Aromatase inhibitors like letrozole in doses of 2.5 mg daily or anastrozole 1 mg daily have been tried in this group of men with promising results. With reduction in peripheral estrogens, not only the semen parameters appear to improve but also the sexual function becomes better in terms of sustained erection and ejaculation. Antiestrogens like clomiphene also find a role in this group of men with variable results.
- *Antioxidants*: Vitamins and minerals are often used in form of antioxidants as empirical first-line therapy for idiopathic mild-to-moderate OATs with variable results. There are reasons for this group of drugs to show little benefit; one of them is that a very small amount of drug crosses the blood testes barrier and the other reason is that only in presence of oxidative stress in semen these drugs may prove to have a role in improving semen parameters by clearing the responsible reactive oxygen species (ROS).

Surgical Management

Varicocele

Surgical correction of varicocele for male infertility has gone through a lot of controversy. However, now it has been established that varicocele repair may be effective in patients who have demonstrable clinical varicocele with abnormal semen parameters and normal female factor. Apart from this, varicocelectomy is also recommended in adolescents if detected early and is found to be progressive in subsequent visits. Surgical intervention may prevent testicular damage and future risk of poor spermatogenesis.

Epididymovasostomy/Vasovasostomy

In men with obstructive azoospermia, these procedures are done microsurgically depending on the site of block. When there is an obstruction at the level of epididymis, epididymovasostomy is required while vasovasostomy is usually done for sterilization reversal. Due to limited success rates of these procedures and development of ART, many clinicians prefer surgical sperm retrieval and IVF with intracytoplasmic sperm injection (ICSI), especially if female partner is of advanced age or low-ovarian reserve.

Surgical sperm retrieval: In patients of azoospermia (obstructive and nonobstructive) surgical sperm retrieval is the next step. These sperm are washed and used for ICSI and can be frozen for future use also. In obstructive azoospermia where surgical correction is not indicated or has failed, sperm can be retrieved from epididymis by percutaneous epididymal sperm aspiration *(PESA)* or microsurgical epididymal sperm aspiration *(MESA)*. The chances of sperm retrieval in these cases are almost 100%. In patients with nonobstructive azoospermia, i.e. testicular failure, there can be foci of spermatogenesis and in approximately 50% of such cases sperm can be found retrieval with testicular sperm aspiration *(TESA)* or testicular sperm extraction *(TESE)*. Microsurgically done procedure *micro-TESE* is known to further improve the chances of sperm retrieval in testicular failure cases.

Assisted reproductive technology—IVF ICSI: All cases of male infertility not amenable to medical or surgical management can now successfully be treated by IVF ICSI including sperms retrieved from testes in cases of azoospermia.

Treatment of Ejaculatory Disorders

Retrograde Ejaculation

This disorder is characterized by low-semen volume with postejaculate urine sample showing sperm, which can be harvested and used.

Anejaculation

Vibrostimulation or electroejaculation can help patients with anejaculation but semen thus obtained is often poor quality and hence IVF ICSI is often required.

Both retrograde ejaculation and anejaculation can be associated with neurological disorders like multiple sclerosis, diabetes mellitus, spinal cord injuries or post-bladder neck or prostate surgery. It is imperative to look into the underlying condition and treat it simultaneously.

UNEXPLAINED INFERTILITY

If all the basic investigations in both partners are normal, the couple is categorized into the group of unexplained infertility. The prevalence of unexplained infertility is very variable and can be as little as 10% to as much as 50% of all cases evaluated for infertility. The incidence depends on how much and with what depth one has tried to investigate the couple to find the cause. Expectant management generally prolongs most in such couples in want of a specific procedure and so does the application of empirical treatment. However, the first-line treatment in couples with unexplained infertility is either the use of ovarian stimulation with IUI and if three to four such cycle of treatment fails to resort to IVF ICSI.

CONCLUSION

- Infertility is defined as inability to conceive after 1 year of regular unprotected intercourse.
- Common causes of infertility include ovulatory disorders (30%), tubal and pelvic pathology (40%), uterine cavity abnormalities (5–10%), and in 20% no cause is found, the so-called unexplained infertility.
- In 20% of infertile couples, male factor is solely responsible for infertility; whereas in another 10–20%, it is present with female factor infertility.
- Initial workup includes tests of ovulation, tubal patency, and semen analysis.
- Depending on the results of couple is categorized into one or more broad groups of infertility such as; tubal factor infertility, ovulatory factor infertility, peritoneal factor or endometriosis or male factor infertility and treated accordingly.
- If all of the above are normal then the couple belongs to the last group of unexplained infertility.
- Treatment of ovulatory disorders is always medical by the help of ovulation inducing agents as first-line treatment; whereas tubal, male factor and unexplained infertility may require the help of ART more often.
- Empirical medicines do not help except for giving a psychological assurance to the couple while awaiting the results with expectant management.

SUGGESTED READING

1. Kamel RM. Management of the infertile couple: an evidence based protocol. Reprod Biol Endocrinol. 2010;8:21.
2. Practice Committee of American Society for Reproductive Medicine. Diagnostic evaluation of infertile female—a committee opinion. Fertil Steril. 2012;98(2):302-7.
3. Practice Committee of American Society of Reproductive Medicine. Diagnostic evaluation of infertile male. Fertil Steril. 2008;90s:178-80.

4. Roux I, Tulandi T, Chan P, et al. Initial investigation of infertile couple. In: Gardner DK, Weissman A, Howles CM, Shoham Z (Eds). Textbook of Assisted Reproductive Techniques: Clinical Perspectives, 4th edition. London: Informa Healthcare; 2012. pp. 31-41.
5. World Health Organization. Report of the Meeting on the Prevention of Infertility at the Primary Health Care Level. Geneva: WHO; 1983, WHO/MCH/1984.
6. World Health Organization. WHO laboratory manual for examination and processing of human semen. Geneva: WHO; 2010.

CHAPTER 13

Contraception: Making the Right Choices

Mamta Dagar

INTRODUCTION

Women's contraceptive choices are largely dependent on advice and counseling from healthcare providers. Efficacy is considered as the most important criteria for opting a contraceptive. Hence, effective communication is vital about the various available methods in a manner, which is acceptable to women in making informed choices.

CONTRACEPTIVE CHOICES AND EFFICACY

Based on their efficacy, contraceptive method can be divided into most effective, effective, and least effective methods (Table 13.1).

How and when to start contraception?

Most contraceptive methods can be initiated on the visit day and require minimum investigations and tests before starting (Table 13.2).

Combined Oral Contraceptive Pills

Combined hormonal contraception offers the widest choice with the best efficacy.

Mechanism of action includes inhibition of ovulation by suppressing luteinizing hormone (LH) and follicle-stimulating hormone (FSH) and alteration of endometrium, which make it unsuitable for implantation.

The tolerability and side effect profile of combined oral contraceptive (COC) has improved since US FDA (Food and Drug Administration) approval in 1960 as the estrogen in the pill has been replaced by ethinylestradiol (EE), and the dose lowered from 150 µg mestranol to 50 and then to 35-20-15 µg EE. The dose of progestin has also been reduced with development of more potent progestins (Table 13.3). Although the third-generation progestins are also derivatives of testosterone, they are more selective with less androgenic activity. A newer progestin, drospirenone (DRSP), a derivative of spironolactone has antiandrogenic and antimineralocorticoid action

Table 13.1: Contraceptive efficacy: 1st year of use.

	Typical use	Perfect use
Most effective		
Intrauterine device	<1	<1
Copper T or Mirena®		
Etonogestrel implant		
Vasectomy		
Effective		
DMPA	6	<1
Contraceptive patch	9	<1
Contraceptive pills		
POP/COCP	9	<1
CVR		
Diaphragm	12	6
Least effective		
Condom		
Male	18	2
Female	21	5
Sponge		
Previous birth	24	20
No previous birth	12	9
Cervical cap (FemCap)		
Previous birth	19	N/A
No previous birth	14	N/A
Fertility awareness-based method		
Cervical mucous or ovulation	24	3
Standards day	24	5
Withdrawal	22	4
Spermicides	28	18
No methods	85	85

(DMPA: depo-medroxyprogesterone acetate; POP: progestin only pill; COCP: combined oral contraceptive pills; CVR: contraceptive vaginal ring)

unlike most other progestogens. The first DRSP containing COC, Yasmin (EE 30 µg/DRSP 3 mg), has hyperkalemia as a potential side effect. A Cochrane Review studied the different progestogens in low-dose COCs and found fewer side effects and consequently lesser discontinuation rates with newer progestogens. DRSP was similar compared to desogestrel regarding contraceptive efficacy, cycle control, and minor side effects.

Contraception: Making the Right Choices

Table 13.2: How to start contraception?

Method	When to start? (Provided there is reasonable certainty that the woman is not pregnant)	Backup method	Tests required before initiating contraception
Cu IUD	Any day of cycle	None	Pelvic examination
LNG IUD	Any day of cycle	If started more than 7 days after menses, abstain for 7 days	Pelvic examination
Implant	Any day of cycle	If started more than 5 days after menses, abstain for 7 days	None
Injectable	Any day of cycle	If started more than 7 days after menses, abstain for 7 days	None
Combined hormonal contraceptive	Any day of cycle	If started more than 5 days after menses, abstain for 7 days	Measurement of BP
POP	Any day of cycle	If started more than 5 days after menses, abstain for 2 days	None

(BP: blood pressure; IUD: intrauterine device; POP: progestin only pill; LNG IUD: levonorgestrel releasing intrauterine device)

Table 13.3: Progestin used in combined oral contraceptive (COC).

Pregnanes	Estranes	Gonanes (Second generation)	Gonanes (Third generation)	Spironolactone analog
Chlormadinone acetate	Norethindrone acetate	DL-norgestrel	Desogestrel	Drospirenone
Cyproterone acetate	Ethynodiol acetate	Levonorgestrel	Gestodene	
Nomegestrol	Lynestrenol		Norgestimate	
Nestorone	Norethynodrel			

The dose of estrogen and progesterone can be same throughout the cycle as in monophasic pills or vary as in multiphasic pills (biphasic, triphasic, and four-phasic) (Table 13.4). The monophasic pill is to be started on day 5 of cycle for 21 days with break of 7 days. Multiple pills have fewer side effects like amenorrhea, breakthrough bleeding, and acne as they aim at reducing the total monthly hormone intake. The drawbacks are compliance issues,

Table 13.4: Constituents of biphasic, triphasic, and four-phasic pills.		
Biphasic pills	Triphasic pills	Four-phasic pills
EE-35 µg constant Low-dose progestin for first 10 days High-dose progestin for next 11 days	EE-3.0 µg constant LNG 0.05 mg for 5 days LNG 0.075 mg for 5 days LNG 0.125 mg for 10 days	E2 (3 mg) + DNG (2 mg) for 2 days. E2 (2 mg) + DNG (2 mg) for 5 days. E2 (2 mg) + DNG (3 mg) for 17 days. E2 (1 mg) + DNG (3 mg) for 2 days.

(E2: estradiol valerate; DNG: dienogest; LNG: levonorgestrel)

increased failure, and difficulty in postponing menses, if needed. Biphasic pills have higher failure rates and are unavailable in India.

Advantages of Qlaira, Four-phasic Pill 2

Fewer spotting days, reduction in mean blood loss, reduced breakthrough bleeding, more increase in high-density lipoprotein (HDL) (8%), stability in carbohydrate mechanism, effective in heavy menstrual bleeding, significant increase in hemoglobin and ferritin levels.

Extended cycle regime has the advantages of decreased incidence of pelvic pain, headaches, bloating, and breast tenderness; improved control over symptoms of endometriosis and polycystic ovarian syndrome; and greater convenience due to fewer withdrawal bleeds per year, however, there is little information on its long-term safety and has slightly higher cost.

Besides the most effective contraceptive efficacy, the noncontraceptive benefits of oral contraceptive pills (OCPs) are listed in Table 13.5.

Progestin-only Pills

Progestin-only oral contraceptives (mini pills) are the best oral contraceptive available for lactating women, as they do not reduce milk production and do not have any estrogenic side effect. The progestin-only pills (POPs) can also be used as emergency contraception after unprotected intercourse. They mainly act by thickening the cervical mucus, suppression of ovulation, and involution of endometrium with efficacy of 99.95%. Various preparations containing progestins-norethindrone, levonorgestrel (LNG), and norgestrel are available. They need to be taken daily without break. Newer Cerazette and Zerogen tablets containing third generation 75 µg Desogestrel have a window period of 12 hours as compared to 3 hours with traditional pills adding to its efficacy.

Table 13.5: Noncontraceptive reproductive benefits of oral contraceptive pill (OCP).

Reduced risk	Reduced risk and improvement of quality of life
Endometrial carcinoma by almost 50%	Dysmenorrhea
Ovarian carcinoma by almost 35%	Menorrhagia
Colorectal carcinoma by almost 40%	Anemia
Benign ovarian cysts	Premenstrual syndrome
Pelvic inflammatory disease	Irregular menses
Ectopic pregnancy	Acne (the newer COC pills)
Benign breast tumors, fibroadenosis decreases by almost 40–70%	Hirsutism (the newer COC pills)
Fibrocystic disease of the breast	Residual protective effect lasts for 10–15 years after stoppage
Preserves bone mineral density after menopause compared to nonusers	

(COC: combined oral contraceptive)

Emergency Contraceptive Pills

Women should be given information about emergency contraception in situations of contraceptive failure. A Cochrane review states that LNG is more effective than the Yuzpe regimen in preventing pregnancy. Single dose (1.5 mg) available with the name Ecee pill, I-pill, Pill 72, administration has similar efficacy as the standard split dose of LNG (0.75 mg) 12 hours apart, to be taken as soon as possible after unprotected intercourse (within 72 hours).

Recently ulipristal acetate (UPA) has been added as a new drug for postcoital contraception. Women with severe cardiovascular diseases, thromboembolic conditions, migraine, and severe liver disorder, and using CYP3A4 inducers can use COCs, LNG, or UPA for emergency contraception (category 2). Women who are breastfeeding can use COCs and LNG as emergency contraceptive pills (ECP) without any restriction (category 1) and UPA as category 2 ECP.

Intrauterine Device: Hormone Releasing

Levonorgestrel-releasing intrauterine device (LNG IUD) 20/Mirena (Fig. 13.1) (LNG IUD) is T-shaped containing 52 mg of LNG polydimethylsiloxane, which releases hormone LNG 20 µg locally daily to maintain the serum progesterone level of 150–200 µg. It is effective for 5 years, with failure rate between 0 and 0.2 per hundred women years.

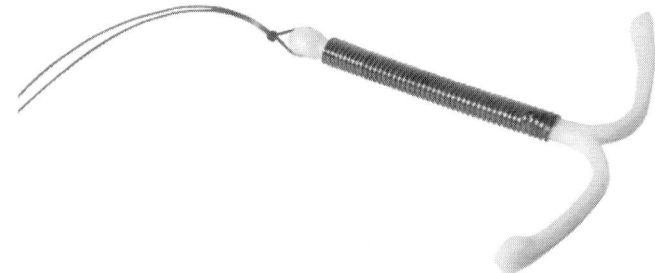

Fig. 13.1: Mirena.

Benefits

- Long-term reversible method
- No daily action needed
- Easy insertion and removal (local anesthesia may be required)
- Lowest dose of hormonal contraceptive with no estrogen
- Reduction in bleeding during menses.

Limitations

- Spotting and intermenstrual bleeding for first few months
- Insertion and removal need trained personnel.

Government of India Initiatives

Centchroman

Among the new entrants in the Government of India basket of choice, which are available to the poorest and to all strata of society are the following contraceptives:
1. *Injection MPA (medroxyprogesterone acetate) under the Antara Program*
2. *Tab Chhaya (Centchroman).*

The above two options, which are very relevant and pertinent in the two most crucial parts of reproductive life of woman, i.e. postpartum and postabortion periods; have already been made available and Delhi is one of the leading states in take up of both these methods.

The injection MPA is a unique suspension of microcrystal for depo injection of pregnant 17-alpha hydroxyprogesterone—a derivative of progestin MPA. The 3 monthly injection is one of the LARC (long-acting reversible contraceptive) option and is given deep intramuscularly in arm, buttock, or thigh. It acts by inhibiting ovulation, thickening of cervical mucus, and thinning of endometrial lining and is as effective as 99.7%.

In other words, its effectiveness surpasses female sterilization, intrauterine contraceptive device (IUCD) and combined oral contraceptive. Being estrogen free, it has an edge over combined oral and injectable methods and can be given almost throughout the reproductive periods to women of any parity and even to breastfeeding women.

The injection also offers many noncontraceptive benefits like reduction in incidence of dysmenorrhea, premenstrual syndrome, anemia, endometriosis, ovarian cyst and cancer, fibroid, benign breast disease, pelvic inflammatory disease (PID), and ectopic pregnancy.

Delayed return to fertility and nonprotection against STI/RTI/HIV are the only limitations besides need to repeat injection every 3 months.

Pill Chhaya (Centchroman): Regarding the second new entrant, which is an oral nonhormonal option, its Government of India brand name is Chhaya and is suitable to many women who want to choose oral but are not fit for hormonal methods. Chemically Chhaya is Centchroman ormeloxifene. The methods are probably one with least limitations, side effects, adverse effects, and contradictions. The first pill is to be taken on the 1st day of period (as indicated by the 1st day of bleeding) and the second pill 3 days later. The pattern of days (biweekly regime) is repeated through the first 3 months. Starting from 4th month, the pill is to be taken once a week on the first pill day and should be continued on the weekly schedule regardless of her menstrual cycle.

The most common side effect (delayed periods), which occurs in 8% of users is to be managed by counseling (both pre and ongoing) and reassurance. Missed pills are managed by taking it as soon as possible after missing (if missed less than 7 days). Additional backup method should also be given. If pills are missed by more than 7 days, client needs to start taking it all over again like a new user, i.e. twice a week for 3 months and then once a week.

Implants

The progestogen only implant is in the form of a single, nonbiodegradable, subdermal rod, 4 cm long and 5 mm in diameter and made of ethylene-vinyl acetate copolymer. It is licensed for up to 3 years of use and contains 68 mg etonogestrel (ENG). The release rate of ENG is 60–70 µg/day in initial 5–6 weeks and 25–30 µg/day at the end of the 3rd year. A bioequivalent implant known as Nexplanon has now replaced Implanon. The main difference is due to barium sulfate, which makes Nexplanon radiopaque. It has a failure rate of 0.05% with side effect of irregular bleeding for first 3–6 months.

Transdermal Delivery Systems

It is available in various forms: patch, gel, and sprays, but only patch is FDA approved. The transdermal combined estrogen/progestin contraceptive patch 20 cm^2 with 600 µg ethinylestradiol (EE) and 6,000 µg norelgestromin releases 20 µg/day of EE + 150 µg/day of norelgestromin. It primarily works by preventing ovulation. Patch can be applied on back, upper arm, abdomen, and buttocks but not the breast. First patch is to be applied on day 1/day 2 of periods and second patch change on the same day of first patch worn. One patch weekly is used consequently for 3 weeks followed by a patch free week. It has a failure rate of 0.7 per 100 women years. Failure is more when body weight is more than 90 kg. Its side effect profile is similar to OCs but is generally well tolerated.

Contraceptive Vaginal Ring

Contraceptive vaginal ring (CVR) is a combined estrogen/progestin contraceptive ring (NuvaRing R), which is flexible and made up of ethylene-vinyl acetate copolymer with 54 mm outer ring diameter and 4 mm of cross-sectional diameter. It releases estrogen (15 μg EE) and progesterone (120 μg Etonogestrel, an active metabolite of Desogestrel) per day. It is used continuously for 3 weeks followed by a gap of 1 week for menstruation to occur. Its insertion and removal are easier, by user's finger. It has contraceptive failure rate of 0.1-0.3 per women years. It should not be kept outside vagina for more than 3 hours.

Copper Intrauterine Device

The mechanism of action of IUDs is by prevention of fertilization and implantation. The duration of action for IUDs containing 380 mm^2 copper lasts between 5 and 10 years and the pregnancy rate associated with it is very low. It is not associated with any delay in the return of fertility following removal or its expulsion.

It may cause heavier bleeding or dysmenorrhea. Majority of women stop using IUDs within 5 years due to increased vaginal bleeding and pain. The risk of uterine perforation at the time of IUD insertion is less than 1 in 1,000, risk of developing pelvic inflammatory diseases is less than 1 in 100. Expulsion rate is less than 1 in 20 women in 5 years. The risk of ectopic pregnancy (about 1 in 1,000 in 5 years) when using IUDs is lower than using no contraception.

Postpartum Intrauterine Contraceptive Devices

Cochrane review concluded that postpartum IUCDs (PPIUCDs) are safe and effective contraceptive method, which can be inserted in the first 48 hours postpartum or 6 weeks following birth.

Male and Female Barrier Methods

As condoms reduced the risk of sexually transmitted infection, their use is recommended in addition to any methods of contraception (Grade 1B) in individual at risk of sexually transmitted disease (STD). Alternative materials to latex rubber include polyurethane and styrene ethylene butylene styrene, which offer advantages over latex condom in terms of a longer shelf life. Polyurethane female condoms (FCI) have been introduced in 1992. The FC2 female condom is made from synthetic latex, which is softer and cheaper than polyurethane. The VA feminine condom, Reddy condom, and V-Amour contain a soft sponge to hold it in place inside the vagina rather than a ring with a higher acceptability than the FCI. The program for approved technology in health (PATH) has developed a woman's condom with a dissolvable capsule to make the insertion easier, a polyurethane condom pouch and a soft outer ring allowing for a nearly universal fit. The SILCS diaphragm fits most women and is more comfortable than existing metal spring devices and can be used with either a spermicide or a lubricant. Overview of contraceptive methods is provided in Table 13.6.

When to stop contraception?

Women who have a copper intrauterine device (Cu-IUD) containing 380 mm^2 copper, inserted at or over the age of 40 years, can retain the device until the menopause or until contraception is no longer required.

Women using nonhormonal methods can be advised to stop contraception after 1 year of amenorrhea (if aged over 50 years and 2 years, if the woman is aged less than 50 years).

Contraception in Medical Disorders

In women with medical disorders, unplanned pregnancy may impose serious risks. Therefore, it is very important to select appropriate method of contraception to avoid unplanned pregnancy.

How to choose the best method of contraception?
- Thorough medical history
- Plans for future pregnancy
- Assess medical eligibility criteria
- Explore the evidence regarding risks, safety, and efficacy
- Consider cost, availability, and acceptability of the contraceptive method.

WHO Medical Eligibility Criteria Wheel (Figs. 13.2A and B)

Barrier contraception can be used for nearly all women and it provides dual advantage of avoiding pregnancy and sexually transmitted infection. The disadvantage is higher failure rate.

Intrauterine contraception device is safe in most medical conditions except in women with complex heart disease, valvular, heart disease, women after kidney transplant where it may be increase chance of infection and in women with anemia where it may be caused increased blood loss. Chances of infection are maximum during the insertion process and can be minimized by taking aseptic precautions. Insertion of IUCD in women with heart disease should be done under anesthesia cover to reduce chances of arrhythmias and vasovagal attacks.

Table 13.6: Overview of contraception methods.

Characteristics	Contraceptive pill, patch or ring	Etonogestrel implant	DMPA	Copper IUD	Levonorgestrel releasing IUD	Male condom	Diaphragm
Pregnancy rate	9	<1	6	<1	<1	18	12
Effective for	pill (use daily), patch (weekly) ring (monthly)	3 years	12 weeks	10 years	3–5 years (depending on type)	Single use	Reusable used with spermicidal
Hormonal exposure	Estrogen and progestin	Progestin	Progestin	—	Progestin	—	—
Effects on menstruation	Lighter, regular, predictable	Lighter, irregular	Lighter, irregular	Heavier	Lighter, irregular first 3–6 months	—	—
Irregular BPV/spotting	Yes	Yes	Yes	Yes	Yes	—	—
Not indicated in	Contraindications to using exogenous estrogen	Poor tolerance of amenorrhea	Irregular bleeding low BMD	HBL anemia, distortion of uterine cavity, active, pelvic infection	Distortion of uterine cavity, active pelvic infection, sensitive to hormonal side effects	Allergy to latex	Allergy to latex, pelvic relaxation
User dependent	Prescription	Yes	Yes	Yes	Yes	Over the counter	Prescription
Selected adverse effects	VTE increased risk of hepatic adenoma	Scarring at insertion/removal site, difficult removal	Weight gain, mood changes, and osteopenia	Uterine perforation expulsion, increased risk of pelvic infection in the first 3 weeks of insertion	Uterine perforation, expulsion, increased risk of pelvic infection in the first 3 weeks of insertion	Condom may break	Urinary tract infection May increase risk

Contd...

Contd...

Characteristics	Contraceptive pill, patch or ring	Etonogestrel implant	DMPA	Copper IUD	Levonorgestrel releasing IUD	Male condom	Diaphragm
Selective advantages	Estrogen benefits—a reduction in dysmenorrhea, menorrhagia, acne, vulgaris, and vasomotor symptoms (peri-menopausal women)	Highly effective	Effective	Highly effective LARC	Reduction in menorrhagia dysmenorrhea and endometrial hyperplasia	Best protection against STI	Low cost and reusable

(BPV: bleeding per vaginum; IUD: intrauterine device; DMPA: depomedroxyprogesterone acetate; HBL: heavy bleeding loss; BMD: bone mineral density; LARC: long-acting reversible contraception; VTE: venous thromboembolism; STI: sexually transmitted infection).
Note: Medical eligibility criteria for contraceptive use WHO MEC, 2015.

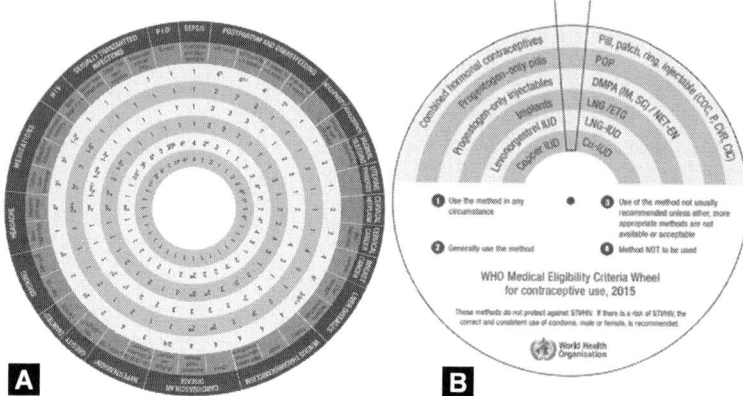

Figs. 13.2A and B: World Health Organization (WHO) Medical Eligibility Criteria (MEC) wheel shown above contains the medical eligibility criteria for starting use of contraceptive methods, based on Medical Eligibility Criteria for contraceptive use, 5th edition (2015), one of WHO evidence-based guidelines.

As estrogen containing contraceptives increase the risk of thrombosis and should be avoided in women with a history of venous thromboembolism, stroke, cardiovascular diseases, or peripheral vascular disease; however, OCPs may be used safely in women in a number of medical disorders like well-controlled hypertension, uncomplicated diabetes mellitus, depression, and uncomplicated valvular heart disease. Women older than 35 years who smoke should avoid OCPs.

Progestin-only contraceptives are recommended for women with contraindication to estrogen and are usually safe in most medical disorders. Desogestrel-containing pills have a positive effect on the course of migraine in majority of women, reducing frequency, analgesics use, and associated symptoms. Injection DMPA is preferred in women with sickle cell disease as it reduces the frequency of painful crisis. It is also favorable for women with antiepilepsy drugs, which induce liver enzymes as it bypasses first pass metabolism (Table 13.7).

Permanent Sterilization

Couple, who desire permanent contraception (sterilization), should also be counseled about vasectomy of the male partner as vasectomy is effective, less morbid but costly than tubal occlusion.

Standards for Female Sterilization

Minilap tubectomy and laparoscopic tubal occlusion are considered safe, acceptable, and simple procedures, which are highly effective and relatively

Table 13.7: Guidelines for prescribing contraceptives in women with medical disorders.

Comorbidity	Methods to consider	Methods to avoid
Depression	COC, DMPA, implant, LNG, IUS, ring, patch, POP	
Diabetes mellitus with complication	DMPA, implant, LNG, IUS, patch, POP	COC, ring, patch
Epilepsy treated with medicines (hepatic enzymes inducers) Carbamazepine, lamotrigine, oxcarbazepine, phenobarbital, phenytoin, primidone, topiramate	DMPA, LNG, IUS	COC, implant, ring, patch, POP
Epilepsy treated without medicine that induce hepatic enzymes Acetazolamide, benzodiazepines, ethosuximide, gabapentin, levetiracetam, pregabalin, tiagabine, valproic acid, vigabatrin, zonisamide	COC, DMPA, implant, LNG, IUS, ring, patch, POP	
History of bariatric surgery (malabsorptive procedure)	COC, DMPA, implant, LNG, IUS, ring, patch	COC, POP
History of bariatric surgery (restrictive procedure)	COC, DMPA, implant, LNG, IUS, ring, patch, POP	—
History of VTE/pulmonary embolism	DMPA, implant, LNG, IUS, POP	COC, ring, patch
Inflammatory bowel disease (mild)	COC, DMPA, implant, LNG, IUS, ring, patch, POP	—
Migraine headaches with aura	DMPA, implant, LNG, IUS, POP	COC, ring, patch
Poorly controlled hypertension	DMPA, implant, LNG, IUS, POP	COC, ring, patch
Rheumatoid arthritis (in patients taking immunosuppressant)	COC, patch, ring, implant, LNG, IUS, POP	DMPA
Smoking and age older than 35	DMPA, implant, LNG, IUS, POP	COC, ring, patch
Stroke	DMPA, implant, LNG, IUS, POP	COC, ring, patch
Systemic lupus erythematosus with antiphospholipid with antibiotics	DMPA, implant, LNG, IUS, POP	COC, ring, patch

(DMPA: depomedroxyprogesterone acetate; LNG: levonorgestrel; COC: combined oral contraceptive; POP: progestin only pills; IUS: intrauterine system)

pain-free. They are inexpensive and suitable to be performed as an ambulatory procedure and cause minimal tubal damage in order to facilitate reversibility. Both methods are considered to be equally safe and effective.

Timing of the Surgical Procedure

Interval sterilization should be performed within 7 days of the onset of menses (in the follicular phase) or anytime during the cycle, if the provider is reasonably certain that the woman is not pregnant. Postpartum sterilization should be performed within 7 days. Sterilization following spontaneous abortion/MTP can be performed concurrently or within 7 days of abortion after excluding infection. It can be performed concurrent with other surgery lower segment cesarean section (LSCS) salpingectomy or ovarian cystectomy.

Eligibility of Clients

Female clients should be more than 22 years and below 49 years. The couple should have at least one child, whose age is more than year. She should be in a sound state of mind, so as to understand the full implications of sterilization. A relevant medical history, physical examination, and laboratory investigations need to be undertaken to ascertain eligibility for surgery.

Laboratory Examination

Test for hemoglobin, urine examination for sugar, and albumin. Pregnancy test is done, if needed. Clients with hemoglobin less than 7 g/dL should not be accepted for sterilization and referred to higher centers for management.

Surgical Procedure

Minilaparotomy

The modified Pomeroy is the recommended approach for occluding the fallopian tubes using a square knot with 1-0 chromic catgut.

Laparoscopic Sterilization

Tubal occlusion must always be done with Falope rings (no cautery is to be used).

CONCLUSION

- Effective communication is vital about the various contraceptive methods in a manner, which is acceptable to women in making informed choices.
- Based on their efficacy, contraceptive method can be divided into Most Effective, Effective and Least Effective methods as combined hormonal contraceptives, Progestin only pills, Intrauterine devices, Injectable Hormonal Contraceptives and Implants and barrier methods.

- Most contraceptive methods can be initiated on the visit day and require minimum investigations and tests before starting.
- In women with medical disorders, it is very important to select an appropriate method of contraception by assessing medical eligibility criteria.
- Couple, who desire permanent contraception, should be counseled about both male and female sterilization methods.

SUGGESTED READING

1. Andrew MK. (2017). Contraceptive counselling and selection. [online] Available from www.uptodate.com. [Accessed November, 2018].
2. Maitra N, Kulier R, Blomenkamp KWM, et al. Progestogens in combined oral contraceptives for contraception (Cochrane Review). The Cochrane Library, Issue 4. Chichester, UK: John Wiley & Sons Ltd; 2004.
3. Medicines and Healthcare products Regulatory Agency (MHRA). (2011). Combined Oral Contraceptives (The Pill): When To Start Taking The Pill And Misses Pill Advice. MHRA UK Public Assessment Report, May 2011. [online] Available from http://www.mhra.gov.uk/safety-public-assessment-reports/CON120481. [Accessed November, 2018].
4. WHO. (2015). World Health Organization MEC for contraceptive use, 5th edition 2015 Executive summary. [online] Available from http://apps.who.int/iris/bitstream/handle/10665/172915/WHO_RHR_15.07_eng.pdf;jsessionid=032A640F7AFF514645BE7668061254A4?sequence=1. [Accessed November, 2018].

CHAPTER 14
Medical Abortion: What a General Practitioner Should Know?

Sharmistha Garg

INTRODUCTION

In view of the rising number of unsafe abortion in the past few years, i.e. from 20 million in 2003 to 22 million in 2008 and the under reported death and morbidity related to this condition, it is necessary to have safe abortion services in our country, so that the physical and mental health of the women can be restored.

The World Health Organization (WHO) defines unsafe abortion as a procedure for terminating an unwanted pregnancy which is carried out either by persons lacking the required skills or in an environment that does not meet even the minimal medical standard or both.

Every year 208 million women are estimated to become pregnant worldwide out of which 59% (123 million) have a planned or intended pregnancy leading to a birth or miscarriage or a still birth. The remaining 41% (or 85 million) of pregnancies are unintended and this is the group of women we are targeting to provide safe abortion services.

Factors that determine the health consequences of unsafe abortions include set up where abortion is performed, the skills of the practitioner, the method of abortion used, woman's health and the gestational age of the pregnancy. Death and disability associated to abortions are difficult to measure due to stigma and fear of punishment which deter reliable reporting of the incident. However, many women do not relate their conditions to a complication of an abortion. Therefore maternal death resulting from unsafe abortions is largely under reported. Complications of unsafe abortions such as sepsis, hemorrhage, peritonitis and trauma to the adjacent organs like cervix, vagina, uterus, and abdominal organs can occur. When medical abortion is provided by skilled practitioner having necessary knowledge and correct medical techniques under aseptic conditions, this procedure becomes very safe.

In the year 1971, the Indian Parliament enacted the Medical Termination of Pregnancy (MTP) Act, with the aim of reducing maternal morbidity and mortality by reducing the incidence of illegal abortion. The MTP Act came into effect from 1 April 1972 and was amended in the years 1975 and 2002.

As per MTP Act pregnancies less than 12 weeks can be terminated on the basis of a single opinion formed in good faith. In case of pregnancies beyond 12 weeks but less than 20 weeks, opinions of two doctors are required for termination. The MTP Act of India clearly states the conditions under which a pregnancy can be ended or aborted, the persons who are qualified to conduct the abortion and the place of implementation. Some of these qualifications are as follows:

- In order to save the life of the pregnant women.
- In order to prevent grave injury to the physical and mental health of the pregnant women.
- In view of the substantial risk that if the child was born it would suffer from such physical or mental abnormalities as to be seriously handicapped.
- As the pregnancy is alleged by pregnant women to have been caused by rape.
- As the pregnancy has occurred as a result of failure of any contraceptive device.

Experience and training required by a Registered Medical Practitioner (RMP) up to 12 weeks gestation (1st trimester): A practitioner who has assisted a RMP in 25 cases of MTP of which at least 5 have been performed independently in a hospital established or maintained by the government or a training institute approved for their purpose by the government.

Up to 20 weeks of gestation (2nd trimester):
- A doctor holding degree or diploma in obstetrics and gynecology.
- A doctor who has completed 6 weeks as house surgeon in obstetrics and gynecology.
- A doctor who has at least 1 year experience in the practice of obstetrics and gynecology at any hospital that has all facilities approved for this purpose by the government.

The Medical Termination of Pregnancy (MTP) Act, 1971 amended in 2002—certain guidelines are:
- MTP can be performed in government institution.
- All the private/voluntary institutions can perform MTP only if they are approved by the district level committee in the districts. No MTP is to be done in any place without registration under MTP Act.
- No MTP is to be done without obtaining consent of the patient in "Form C" as per MTP Act. For "minors" or "mentally ill" patients, consent of the guardians is to be taken in "Form C".
- For MTP up to 1st trimester up to 12 weeks, opinion of one RMP and for 2nd trimester pregnancy, opinion of 2 RMPs is to be taken in "Form 1".

- For all MTP cases, admission register as per format of "Form III" under the MTP Act is to be maintained which should be kept in secret custody. Reference to the woman in other records will be made by serial number assigned to her in the admission register.
- Under the Act, MTP is performed under specific selective reasons. Sex selection is not one of the indications for MTP. Hence, no MTP is to be done for sex selection purpose which is prohibited and punishable under the Act.

Various forms and records to be maintained as per Government of India MTP Act, 1971:

Form A: Application form for site approval

Form B: Certificate of approval

Form C: Consent form

Form I: Opinion form of RMP with list of indications for MTP

Form II: MTP reporting form

Form III: Admission registers with 14 columns:

- Monthly report with regard to the MTP performance as per "Form III" is to be submitted by each center of DFWB/district authorities on the 1st day of every month. 100% collection of MTP reports both from government/private institutions is to be ensured by the DFWB of each district.
- Original MTP registration certificate is to be displayed in waiting area of the approved hospital.

Recently, a rape survivor was permitted to terminate her 24-week-old pregnancy according to the ruling by the Supreme Court, which is beyond the permissible 20 weeks limit prescribed under the MTP Act, 1971.

An adult woman requires no other person's consent except her own.

FORM C
(See rule 8)

I_____
daughter/wife of _____
___aged about _____ years of _____
_____
(Here state the permanent address) at present residing at _____
_____ do hereby give my
consent to the termination of my pregnancy at_____
_____
_____
_____

(State the name of place where the pregnancy is to be terminated)

Place:

Date: Signature

(To be filled in by guardian where the woman is a *mentally ill person* or minor)
I_____ son/daughter/wife of
_____
aged about _____
years of _____ at present residing
at (Permanent address) _____
_____
_____ do hereby give my consent to the termination of the pregnancy
of my ward _____ who
is a minor/lunatic at _____
(Place of termination of my pregnancy)

Place:

Date: Signature

Form I
(See Regulation 3)

I_____
(Name and qualifications of the Registered Medical Practitioner in block letters)

_____
(Full address of the Registered Medical Practitioner)

I_____
(Name and qualifications of the Registered Medical Practitioner in block letters)

_____
(Full address of the Registered Medical Practitioner) hereby certify that *I/We am/are of opinion, formed in good faith, that it is necessary to terminate the pregnancy of _____

_____
(Full name of pregnant woman in block letters) resident of _____ _____ (Full address of pregnant woman in block letters) for the reasons given below.**

*I/We hereby give intimation that *I/We terminated the pregnancy of the women referred to above who bears the serial No. _____
in the Admission Register of the hospital/approved place.

Place_____ Signature of the Registered Medical Practitioner

Date_____ Signature of the Registered Medical Practitioners

Strike out whichever is not applicable.

**of the reasons specified items (i) to (v) write the one which is appropriate:

(i) in order to save the life of the pregenent woman.
(ii) in order to prevent grave injury to the physical and mental health of the pregnant woman.
(iii) in view of the substantial risk that if the child was born it would suffer from such physical or mental abnormalities as to be seriously handicapped.
(iv) as the pregnancy is alleged by pregnant woman to have been caused by rape.
(v) as the pregnancy has occurred as result of failure of any contraceptive device or methods used by married woman or her husband for the purpose of limiting the number of children.

Note: Account may be taken of the pregnant woman's actual or reasonably foresseable environment in determining whether the continuance of her pregnancy would involve a grave injury to her physical or mental health.

Place_____   Signature of the Registered
                                              Medical Practitioner

For more information kindly refer to MTP Act, 1971 (Government of India guidelines).

CLINICAL CARE OF THE WOMEN UNDERGOING ABORTIONS
Preabortion Care
- First, the pregnancy has to be confirmed and, if so, the duration of pregnancy should be calculated and confirm that pregnancy is intrauterine.
- Proper history taking is important which includes confirming the first day of last menstrual period (LMP), duration and amount of bleeding and regularity of cycles. Lactating women may become pregnant even before their first postpartum menses. Similarly women using injectable hormonal contraception may become pregnant after missing an injection. Some women may experience slight spotting in early pregnancy and this can be a cause of missing or misdating pregnancy.
- Personal and family history of any medical disorder like hypertension, diabetes, coagulopathies, obstetric and gynecologic history including previous ectopic pregnancy, history of presence of sexually transmitted disease should be taken. Current use of any medications, known allergies and risk of assessment of violence should be done.
- *Physical examination*:
    - Includes pulse, blood pressure, and temperature
    - Confirm pregnancy by bimanual examination
    - Rule out ectopic pregnancy if uterus is less than dates, any tenderness on bimanual examination
    - Rule out condition like sexually transmitted diseases and anemia.
- *Laboratory testing*: ABO, Rh typing, hematocrit should be done. However laboratory testing is not prerequisite for abortions unless typical signs of pregnancy are not present.
- *Ultrasound screening*: Not routinely required for abortion but in centers where facilities are available it can be done to confirm site, viability, age, number of sac, and to rule out ectopic and molar pregnancy.
- *Role of antibiotic*: Routine use of antibiotic for medical abortion is not recommended. However, reproductive tract infections should be ruled out and necessary antibiotic prophylaxis should be given in such cases.
- *Ectopic pregnancy*:
    - Occurs in 1.5–2% of pregnancies.
    - Ectopic pregnancy is presence of gestational sac anywhere outside the uterine cavity, i.e. fallopian tube, ovaries, abdominal or cervical.
    - It should always be ruled out before prescribing medical abortion by high degree of suspicion in cases where uterus is smaller than dates, cervical motion tenderness, adnexal mass, history of vaginal bleeding. In every cases history of missing the period may not be there.
- Rh immunization must be given in cases of Rh negative nonimmunized pregnancy.

- *Information and counseling*: Women should be provided information for various methods of abortions, the effects and complications of each method, follow-up care and contraception care after that.

MEDICAL METHODS OF ABORTION: ADAPTED FROM WORLD HEALTH ORGANIZATION SAFE ABORTION GUIDELINES 2012

> **Box 14.1:** Medical methods of abortion—adapted from World Health Organization Safe Abortion Guidelines 2012.
>
> *Mifepristone followed by misoprostol are the recommended drugs for medical abortion:*
>
> *For pregnancies of gestational age up to 9 weeks (63 days)*: The recommended method of medical abortion is mifepristone followed by misoprostol administered 24–48 hours later.
>
> *Dosages and routes of administration for mifepristone followed by misoprostol*: Mifepristone should always be administered orally. The recommended dose is 200 mg. Administration of misoprostol is recommended 24–48 hours following ingestion of mifepristone.
> - The recommended dose of misoprostol is 800 µg for vaginal, buccal or sublingual routes.
> - The recommended dose of misoprostol is 400 µg for oral administration.
> - Up to 7 weeks (49 days) of gestation misoprostol may be administered by vaginal, buccal, sublingual or oral routes. After 7 weeks of gestation, oral administration of misoprostol is not recommended.
> - Up to 9 weeks (63 days) of gestation misoprostol can be administered by vaginal, buccal or sublingual routes.
>
> *For pregnancies between 9–12 weeks (63–84 days) gestation*: The recommended dose is 200 mg mifepristone to be given orally followed by 800 µg of misoprostol to be given vaginally, 36–48 hours later. Subsequent misoprostol doses should be 400 µg, to be given either vaginally or sublingually, every 3 hours up to four further doses, until expulsion of the products of conception.
>
> *For pregnancies of gestational age more than 12 weeks (84 days)*: The recommended dose for medical abortion is 200 mg mifepristone to be given orally followed by repeated dose of misoprostol 36–48 hours later.
> - With gestation between 12 and 24 weeks, the initial misoprostol dose following oral mifepristone administration may be either 800 µg administered vaginally or 400 µg administered orally. Subsequent misoprostol doses should be 400 µg, every 3 hours up to four further doses administered either sublingually or vaginally.
> - For pregnancies between 12 and 24 weeks, mifepristone followed by 800 µg of misoprostol to be given 3 hourly up to four further doses.
>
> Where mifepristone is not available?
>
> *For pregnancies of gestational age less than 12 weeks (84 days)*: The recommended dose for medical abortion is 800 µg of misoprostol to be given vaginally or sublingually. Up to three repeat doses of 800 µg can be given at intervals of at least 3 hours but for no longer than 12 hours.
>
> Where mifepristone is not available?
>
> *For pregnancies of gestational age more than 12 weeks (84 days)*: The recommended method of medical abortion is 400 µg of misoprostol administered vaginally or sub lingually, repeated every 3 hours for up to five doses.

COMPLICATIONS OF ABORTIONS

- *Ongoing pregnancy*: Women with ongoing symptoms of pregnancy or clinical signs of failed abortion should be offered uterus evacuation as soon as possible.
- *Incomplete abortion*: Symptoms include vaginal bleeding and abdominal pain. Management depends on clinical condition of women, amount of blood loss and her preference. Repeat dose of Misoprostol 400-600 µg through nonvaginal route can be given or immediate vacuum evacuation should be offered.
- *Hemorrhage*: It can be due to reduced products of conception, uterine perforation, coagulopathy and the treatment depends on the cause.
- *Infections*: Common presenting symptoms include fever with chills, foul smelling vaginal or cervical discharge, abdominal, and pelvic pain. Prolong vaginal bleeding or spotting, uterine tenderness, elevated white blood cells count.

Postabortion Care

It is required to protect the woman from morbidity and mortality related to complications of abortion including incomplete evacuation. Continuous heavy bleeding with or without passage of clots should draw attention of physician to offer the patient surgical evacuation. Contraception counseling after abortion is very necessary including emergency contraception as the couple is more receptive to the advice and more likely to follow it also. Details of type of contraceptive methods are explained in another chapter on contraception later on in this book. Postabortal hormonal contraception can be prescribed immediately if patient is not breastfeeding. Cervical caps and diaphragms are contraindicated immediately after abortion. Intrauterine devices can be inserted after abortion once uterine evacuation is complete, however rate of expulsion is high after second trimester abortion. Proper information should also be provided against infection prevention, i.e. STDs so in patients with history of multiple partners use of condom should be encouraged.

CONCLUSION

- The National Center for Health Statistics, the Centers for Disease Control and Prevention and the WHO defines abortion as termination of pregnancy before 20 weeks gestation or fetal weight less than 500 g.
- Safe abortion is a right of every woman and it is our duty to provide them.
- Confirm pregnancy, its duration and site before prescribing medical abortion.
- Proper information of various methods available, effects, complication should be explained to them.

- Informed consent is mandatory as per MTP Act, 1971 before prescribing medical abortion.
- Patient should be given information about when to report to hospital like heavy bleeding per vaginum, fainting attacks, high-grade fever.

SUGGESTED READING

1. Ministry of Health and Family Welfare. (2016). The Medical Termination of Pregnancy Act, 1971. [online]. Available from https://mohfw.gov.in/acts-rules-and-standards-health-sector/acts/mtp-act-1971 [Accessed November, 2018].
2. WHO. (2012). Safe Abortion Practices Guidelines. [online]. Available from http://apps.who.int/iris/bitstream/handle/10665/97415/9789241548717_eng.pdf;jsessionid=7BC20D5D312FED6A274E48D84C6B85A8?sequence=1 [Accessed November, 2018].

CHAPTER

15

Breast Cancer Surveillance

Debasis Dutta, Kanika Chopra

INTRODUCTION

Breast diseases represent a very wide variety of pathological entities, at one end of the spectrum, there are benign forms like fibroadenomas, fibrocystic disease extending to various malignancies. Women's healthcare provider should understand the evaluation and treatment of breast lesion as only 6% of cases present with mass. The gynecologists are usually the first encounter; a woman consults for breast diseases and also for other genital tract-related conditions. So, it is the responsibility of the consulting doctor to examine the patient completely and take it as an opportunity to teach her the importance of self-breast examination and go on to further need for investigation and referral to breast oncologist if the need arises. The differences in palpable consistencies and radiographic density between gland and fat, makes it a challenging task, so one has to be very vigilant and ensure proper screening of breast tumors.

BREAST ANATOMY (FIG. 15.1)

Female breast is a modified sebaceous gland resting on the superficial fascia of chest wall and breast in totality is made of 12–20 lobules, glands, milk ducts, connective tissue, and fat. In younger patients, breast consists mainly of glandular tissue and this is with age replaced by fat. Glandular component of the breast is highly sensitive to estrogen along with the growth of adipose tissue and lactiferous ducts. Progesterone on the other hand, leads to the growth of lobules and alveolar budding.

PATIENTS HISTORY AND PHYSICAL EXAMINATION

Patient may present with complaints of breast pain, mass or nipple discharge. So, it is important to take a look at all the symptoms carefully and enquire about its onset and rate of progression. Also, one has to look into the presence of risk factors as well, including positive family history. Complete breasts

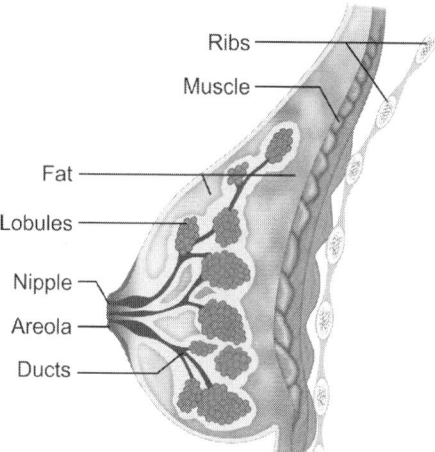

Fig. 15.1: Breast anatomy.

examination during follicular phase of menstrual cycle should then be done, in a systemic fashion, including complete chest wall and both the axillae. The features suggestive of malignancy in a breast mass are size more than 2 cm, immobility of the mass, poorly defined margins, firmness, skin dimpling, color changes, retraction or change in nipple size, bloody discharge from nipple, and lymphadenopathy.

Factors regarded as high risk for breast cancer:
- *Age*: Risk of breast cancer increases exponentially with age, rising steadily after 50 years, approximately 1.4% between 40 years and 49 years and 3.7% between 60 years and 69 years.
- *Race*: Breast cancer is more commonly seen in white women and those of Jewish heritage.
- *Family history*: There is a strong positive correlation between ovarian and breast cancer at an early age in first-degree relatives.
- *Genetics*: Patient having BRCA1 and BRCA2 mutations.
- *Reproductive and menstrual history*: Early menarche and continuation of menstrual periods after the age of 55 years are at a high risk of breast malignancy. Nulliparity and late age at first child and not breastfeeding, adds on to the risk.
- *Radiation exposure*: In patients, who underwent radiotherapy for Hodgkin's disease and enlarged thymus, falls under the high-risk category for breast cancer. The cumulative dose of less than 20 cGy does not cause any significant damage.
- *Breast changes*: Presence of dense breast tissue, atypical hyperplasia, and lobular carcinoma in situ.
- *Other factors*: Overweight, alcohol consumption.

TYPES OF LESIONS IN BREAST

Nonproliferative Lesions

A wide variety of fibrocystic changes in the breast are quite common. Simple fibroadenoma among these changes is usually found in late teens and early twenties. It is described as a solid, round, and mobile mass. These usually respond to conservative management. Others common lesions are lactational adenomas and cysts, fibrosis, and adenosis.

Proliferative Changes with No Atypia

Lesions which present as palpable mass but not detected by mammography are epithelial hyperplasia, sclerosing adenosis, complex sclerosing lesions, and papillomas.

Proliferative Lesions with Atypia

Lesions like lobular and ductal carcinoma in situ can only be definitively diagnosed by excisional biopsy. However, preventive therapy with selective estrogen receptor modulators (SERMs) like tamoxifen should be instituted prior to procedure to prevent the risk of invasive cancer (Table 15.1).

BREAST CANCER

In women among the various malignancies, breast cancer is quite common. Incidence of breast cancer is on the rise, which may be due to increased detection by mammography.

Gail Model: Breast Cancer Risk Assessment Tool

The Gail Model developed by the National Cancer Institute enumerate eight risk factors as predictors for developing breast cancer which are as follows:

Table 15.1: Pathologic lesions of breast.

Pathologic lesions	Fibrocystic changes	Risk of developing invasive breast cancer
Nonproliferative	• Cysts, fibrosis, and adenosis • Lactational adenomas • Fibroadenomas	1.0
Proliferative lesions without atypia	• Sclerosing adenosis • Epithelial hyperplasia • Papillomas • Complex sclerosing lesions	1.5–2.0
Proliferative with atypia	• In situ lobular cancers • In situ ductal cancers	8.0–10.0

1. Race
2. Ethnic background
3. Age
4. Age of menarche
5. Age at which first live baby born
6. Number of first-degree relative with breast cancer
7. History of breast biopsy
8. History of lobular carcinoma in situ (LCIS), ductal carcinoma in situ (DCIS).

This tool is sensitive to estimate the risk of breast cancer over the next 5 years, till 90 years of age. Women with a 5-year survival risk of 1.7% or more can be referred for possible prophylactic therapy which includes chemoprevention with SERMs like tamoxifen and raloxifene, and prophylactic mastectomy.

Histological Types of Breast Cancers

All the major components of the breast tissue are at the risk of developing malignancies and accordingly, they are histologically categorized into ductal, lobular, and cancers of the nipple. Ductal carcinomas are the most common seen in 70–80% of cases and they have mostly spread by lymphatic route to regional lymph nodes. Next common cancers are lobular cancers comprising of 5–50% of all breast cancers and are often multifocal in origin involving both breasts.

Paget diseases involving nipple are rare and simulates skin eczema.

Surgical staging helps in deciding extent of surgery, as per the TNM system suggested by the American Joint Committee on Cancer stages breast malignancies of TNM system. The next thing important is the receptor status. Estrogen and progesterone receptor positivity is correlated directly with good prognosis. On the other hand, overexpression of human epidermal growth factor receptor 2 (HER2)/neu receptor is associated with unfavorable prognosis.

Breast Cancer Treatment

The surgical treatment offered is either lumpectomy or mastectomy. The main aim of the procedure is to achieve local control. Radiotherapy is used in combination with mastectomy in patients with advanced stage, and after lumpectomy for early stages of cancer.

Adjuvant systemic therapy with SERMs like tamoxifen and raloxifene are used in all stages of breast cancer management. In addition, aromatase inhibitors are used to decrease the production of estrogen in the postmenopausal women.

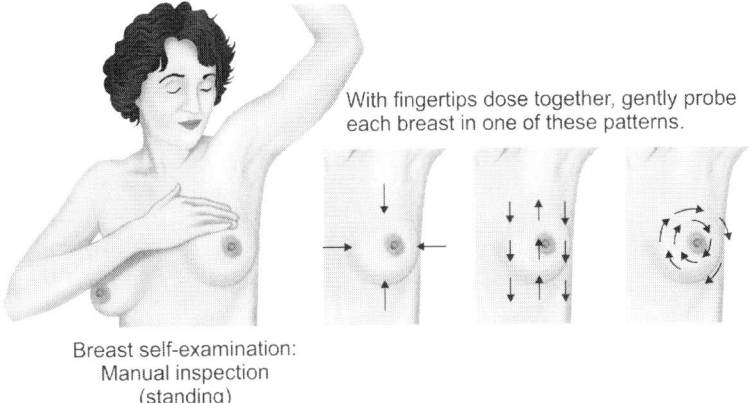

Fig. 15.2: Self-breast examination.

Screening of Breast Cancer

- *Self-breast examination*: Self-breast examination is done every month after menstrual cycle. The patient unclothes herself and sits in front of a mirror and examines her breast completely (Fig. 15.2). The various maneuvers are hands by the side, hands pressed against the hips, hands above the head, and stooping forward. She has to palpate her both breasts with the palmar surface of the hand and also press the areolar region to look for any nipple discharge. The female is taught to look for changes in size, contour, nipple retraction, elevation, lumps, and skin changes like erythema, dimpling, and ecchymosis. All women should be taught self-breast examination by the age of 20 years.
- *Self and clinical assessment*: Clinical and self-breast examination; only difference is that it is performed by the clinician. Obstetricians and gynecologists should take it as an opportunity for breast examination.
- *Mammography*: This modality is an advancement which helps in early detection of nonpalpable lesions approximately 2 years before they become palpable. It is considered as the first-line modality in evaluating a patient after 40 years of age. Advancement in the technology has drastically improved the mammography images and also reduced the radiation dose. Significant decrease in mortality due to breast cancer has been noted after inception of mammography. It is, thus, referred as the most potent weapon in battle against breast cancer as it helps in decreasing both mortality as well as morbidity. About 10% of mammography requires additional evaluation, due to difficulty in achieving accurate mammography in young patients because of denser, more glandular breasts in younger women.
- Advantage of mammography is that it can be used both as screening as well as a diagnostic tool. In clinically apparent mass, bilateral

mammography is done. The images are evaluated for defects which can be suspicious of malignancy and includes microcalcification, discrete nonpalpable lesions, and distortion of normal architecture. Lobular cancers are usually difficult to be detected.

The Breast Imaging Reporting and Data System (BIRADS) is standardization of reporting of mammographic results devices by the American College of Radiology along with the National Cancer Institute and the Food and Drug Administration (FDA). *It clearly communicates the final assessment and recommendation to the treating physician* (Table 15.2).

Digital mammography is superior to routine mammography in younger patients with dense breasts. Its advantages are easier access to images with more efficient storage of images, the use of computer-aided reading of images, and even rapid data transfer between clinical settings.

- *Ultrasonography*: Ultrasonography can detect lesions not seen by mammography.

Women with dense breast are at an increased risk of developing breast cancer; ultrasonography is a better modality and thus, improves the sensitivity of screening. In patients with less than 40 years of age, it is used as an initial screening modality. American College of Radiology Imaging Network (ACRIN) 6,666 trial defined false-positive rate for mammography as 4.4%, for ultrasound as 8.1%, and that of combined detection with ultrasound and mammography as 10.4%. It also revealed that adding ultrasound to mammography leads to detection of additional 4.2 cancers per 1,000 high-risk woman.

Table 15.2: The Breast Imaging Reporting and Data System (BIRADS).

BIRADS classification	Summary recommendation	Explanation
0	Needs additional imaging evaluation	A mammogram with a lesion which needs additional imaging
1	Negative	Breast appears normal
2	Benign findings	Negative mammogram but interpreter wishes to describe a finding
3	Probable benign findings	A mammogram with a lesion high likely to be benign. Follow-up suggested.
4	Suspicious abnormality	A concerning lesion with a definite probability of being malignant, biopsy recommended
5	Highly suspicious of malignancy	A lesion with a high probability of being cancer—appropriate referral to a breast oncologist required
6	Known biopsy proven	Appropriate action should be taken

- *Magnetic resonance imaging*: The most sensitive technique tool to detect breast lesions suggestive of malignancy is MRI. It can even detect DCIS, not detected by mammography and even ultrasonography. The only disadvantage of this procedure is that, it is expensive and intravenous injection of contrast which is poorly tolerated by many patients.
- *Fine-needle aspiration biopsy (FNAB)*: It is a technique very useful in detecting if a palpable lump is a simple cyst or not. FNAB is carried as an office procedure under local anesthesia using 22-24 gauge needle. If clear fluid is aspirated, nothing need to be done aggressively if the breast mass disappears except routine evaluation. If bloody fluid is aspirated, it requires pathological evaluation and further mammography along with ultrasound for better evaluation.
- *Core needle biopsy*: It is done using a 14-16 gauze needle to obtain samples from large and solid masses. These samples are then evaluated for the presence of abnormal cells in relation with surrounding normal breast cells.

Triple approach defined as breast examination, mammography, possibly ultrasound in young women, and needle aspiration helps in a better detection of breast malignancy with at least one of the three diagnostic tests. Open biopsy can, thus, be best avoided (Table 15.3).

Table 15.3: Breast Cancer Screening Guidelines for women.

Age groups	US Preventive Task Force, 2016	American Cancer Society, 2015	American College of Obstetricians and Gynecologists, 2011
40–49 years with average risk	The women may choose to begin biennial screening between 40 years and 49 years of age, but the decision should be on the individual herself	Yearly mammogram is advocated for women aged 45–49 years, however, they should be given the choice to choose their screening program	Screening with mammography and clinical breast examination annually
50–74 years with average risk	Biennial screening mammography	▪ Yearly mammogram is suggested for women aged 50–54 years ▪ 2-yearly mammogram is suggested after that and the women should be given the choice to continue screening program	Screening with mammography and clinical breast examination annually

Contd...

Contd...

Age groups	US Preventive Task Force, 2016	American Cancer Society, 2015	American College of Obstetricians and Gynecologists, 2011
Women with average risk more than 75 years of age	In women more than 75 years of age, there is presently insufficient evidence to assess the balance between benefits and harms of screening mammography	Continue screening till women in good health	Women in association with their physician and should decide whether to continue screening or not
Women with dense breast	At present, there is insufficient evidence to assess the balance between benefits and harms of adjunctive screening for breast cancer using breast ultrasonography or MRI, in women who have dense breast, or otherwise negative screening mammograms	There is limited evidence to recommend for or against yearly MRI screening	Limited evidence exists to recommend for or against MRI screening
Women with higher than average risk for breast cancer	Starting screening at 40 years benefits women at a higher risk for breast cancer	Yearly mammogram is advocated for women with first-degree relative having BRCA1 or BRCA2 mutations	<ul><li>Twice yearly clinical breast examination, annual mammography, annual breast MRI, and self-breast examination is suggested for women who test positive for BRCA1, BRCA2 mutations or they have a lifetime risk of 20% or greater risk to develop the disease.</li><li>Woman recipient of thoracic radiation between 10 years and 30 years of age should undergo annual</li></ul>

Contd...

Contd...

Age groups	US Preventive Task Force, 2016	American Cancer Society, 2015	American College of Obstetricians and Gynecologists, 2011
			mammography, annual MRI, and screening clinical breast examination every 6–12 months beginning 8–10 years after radiation treatment or at the age of 25 years
Additional issues relevant for all women	There is insufficient current evidence to conclude whether digital tomosynthesis, as a primary screening method for breast cancer, is harmful or beneficial	Women should be familiar with the known benefits, limitations, and potential harms associated with breast cancer screening. They should also be familiar with how their breast normally look and feel and report any changes to a healthcare provider as soon as possible	Not addressed

CONCLUSION

- Women with average risk and of the age 40–74 years should have annual clinical breast examination done along with mammography.
- Women aged more than 75 years can decide whether to continue mammographic screening in consultation with their clinician.
- For women who test positive for BRCA1 or BRCA2 mutations or have a lifetime risk of 20% or greater, screening should include twice yearly clinical breast examinations, annual mammography, annual bra breast MRI, and self-breast examination.

SUGGESTED READING

1. American College of Obstetrician-Gynecologists. Practice bulletin no. 122: Breast cancer screening. Obstet Gynecol. 2011;118(2 Pt 1):372-82.
2. Oeffinger KC, Fontham ET, Etzioni R, et al. Breast Cancer Screening for Women at Average Risk: 2015 Guideline Update From the American Cancer Society. JAMA. 2015;314(15):1599-614.
3. Siu AL, US Preventive Services Task Force. Screening for Breast Cancer: US Preventive Services Task Force Recommendation Statement. Ann Intern Med. 2016;164(4): 279-96.

CHAPTER 16

Screening of Gynecological Cancers

Indrani Ganguli

INTRODUCTION

Cancers affecting the female reproductive system are known as gynecological cancers. Cervical, ovarian, vaginal, vulvar, endometrial or uterine, tubal cancers, and breast cancer are different types of gynecological cancer. Like other cancers, gynecological cancers are multifactorial disease characterized by uncontrolled division and growth of the cells. Cancerous cells have unique property to migrate and invade other organs. This uncontrolled cell division and growth are attributed to both cellular and environmental factors.

Incidence of gynecological cancers in women is quite high. Intensive research work is being carried out worldwide as well as in India to understand the molecular mechanism of cancer development. Various screening procedure and treatment modalities are also available. With current advancement of science and technology cancers can be eradicated completely, if the diagnosis is made in early stage of disease. In developing countries like India, diagnosis is usually made at advance stage of the disease, making the treatment difficult.

Screening is defined as use of a test or a combination of tests for an asymptomatic population who are at risk of developing the disease at an earlier and more curable stage. Screening is the potential way to improve the outcome. It detects cancer at an early stage when the prognosis is good. It is very important to counsel the patients undergoing cancer screening as the false-positive and false-negative results are possible. The screening procedures are not flawless.

There are certain established set of principles to guide the development of screening procedure by World Health Organization (WHO).
- The disease should pose an important health problem.
- The natural history or progression of the disease should be well understood.
- There should be a recognizable early stage of the disease.

- Treatment of the disease at an early stage should be of more beneficial than if the treatment is delayed.
- There must be a suitable test available.
- The screening procedure should be acceptable to the population.
- There should be adequate facilities for the diagnosis and treatment.
- Disease of insidious onset screening should be repeated at regular intervals.
- Cost of screening should be balanced against benefits.
- Chance of physical or psychological harm should be less than the benefit.

Among various gynecological cancers, progression of disease and preinvasive lesion are well-established in cervical cancer. Hence, it is more amenable for screening. In case of uterine cancer, the patient is symptomatic in early stage of the disease. Whereas progression of disease and preinvasive lesion are not well established for tubal, ovarian, vulval, and vaginal cancer.

In this chapter, the screening procedure of various gynecological cancers and how these procedures will help the women to fight against cancer will be discussed.

CERVICAL CANCER

Lower part of uterus or womb is known as cervix, which is again divided into ectocervix and endocervix. Ectocervix is covered by squamous epithelium and lining of the endocervix is made by the glandular cells. Malignancy of cervix is known as cervical cancer.

Cervical cancer is the third most common gynecological cancer worldwide. In 2012, 528,000 new cases have been reported along with 266,000 deaths. Its incidence rate is higher in developing countries compared to the developed region of the world.

Risk Factors of Cervical Cancer

Human papillomavirus (HPV) is the central cause of cervical cancer and is detected in 99.7% of cases. There are various subtypes of HPV. Among them, approximately 15 subtypes are oncogenic in nature and subtype 15 and 16 are found in 70% of all cervical cancer cases. With the discovery of HPV vaccine, there is expectation in reduction in rate of HPV infection and as a result reducing the incidence of cervical cancer. There is declining trend of incidence of cervical cancer in developed countries due to availability of screening procedures and vaccination.

Other risk factors include multiple sexual partners, early sexual debut, first full-term baby below the age of 17, multiparity and unhygienic living conditions.

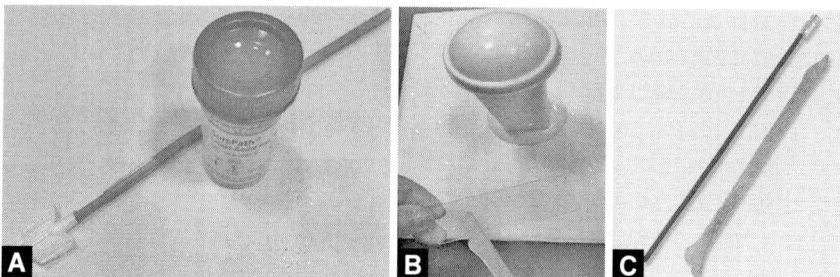

Figs. 16.1A to C: Liquid-based cytology (LBC) and Pap smear.

Screening

Screening detects cervical cancer in precancerous stage, which gives 100% survival rate after proper treatment. Screening of cervical cancer is usually done by cervical cytology (by Pap smear or by liquid-based cytology method) and test for HPV.

In Pap smear, cells are collected during speculum examination by a brush or spatula followed by spreading over a slide. Finally, the slide is dipped in preservative. In liquid-based cytology, the cells are collected by the brush and directly transferred to preservative liquid (Figs. 16.1A to C). The final examination is performed by cytopathologists under a microscope.

Problems Associated with Sampling

Sample cannot be collected during menstruation. On the day of sampling, the concerned person should not use any vaginal medicine or douche. The person should not have sexual intercourse on the night before the day of sampling.

Frequency of Screening

Between the age of 21 years and 65 years, Pap smear or liquid cytology test should be performed every 3 years, whereas the HPV testing along with cytology is recommended every 5 years.

At age more than 65, screening is not required, if the person has been screened enough in her reproductive life. However, if the person has ever undergone any precancerous treatment, screening is recommended for another 20 years even if the person is older than 65 years. Persons having uterus removed for a noncancerous condition do not need screening for cervical cancer.

What is abnormal?
Presence of atypical squamous cells of undetermined significance (ASCUS), low-grade squamous intraepithelial lesion (LSIL), high-grade squamous

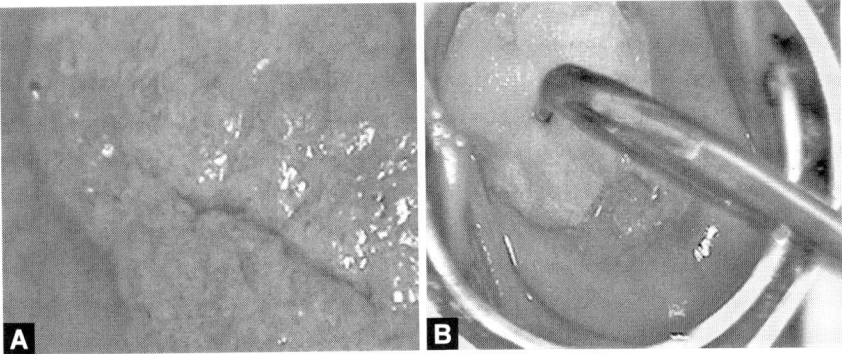

Figs. 16.2A and B: Colposcopy.

intraepithelial lesion (HSIL), and atypical glandular cells of undetermined significance (AGUS) are referred as abnormality found in screening.

What to do if the cytology report is abnormal?
If ASCUS is detected in cytology test, follow-up after 6 months is recommended. If the result is abnormal even after 6 months then colposcopy directed biopsy is recommended. For LSIL, HSIL, and AGUS, colposcopy-directed biopsy should be advised irrespective of HPV status (Figs. 16.2A and B).

BREAST CANCER

Tata Memorial Hospital reported cervical cancer is the most frequent gynecological cancer in India. However, in three metropolitan cities of India namely Delhi, Mumbai, and Kolkata, breast cancer is most prevalent gynecological cancer. It mainly affects females, though 1% of male population also develop breast cancer.

Risk Factors

The risk factors of breast cancer include:
- Family history of breast cancer
- Family history of other gynecological cancers
- Late menarche or early menopause
- Taking hormone therapy including oral contraceptive pills
- High-fat diet
- Smoking and drinking alcohol
- Positive *BRCA1* and *BRCA2* gene mutation.

Genetic Predisposition to Breast Cancer

In approximately 5–10% of all breast cancer are genetically predisposed. Mutations in *BRCA1* and *BRCA2* genes increase the risk of developing breast and ovarian cancer. *BRCA*-related breast cancers are associated with more severe phenotypes than the sporadic cases. Various studies have established significant association of *BRCA* related breast cancer with triple negative phenotype (negative for estrogen and progesterone receptors and reduced expression of *HER2*). Apart from *BRCA* genes, germline mutations in *PTEN*, *TP53*, *CDH1*, and *STK11* genes also increase the risk of developing breast cancer. These germline mutations can easily be detected by genetic testing, which help in better management of the disease.

Screening

There are various ways to screen breast cancer. Some of them are as follows:
- Self-examination of the breast
- Examination by a clinician
- Mammography
- Magnetic resonance imaging (MRI)
- Examination by ultrasound
- Screening for presence of genetic mutation
- Various modern image-based techniques.

Self-examination of Breast

The breast must be examined postmenstrual and every month on the same day of every month. Palpation of upper and outer quadrant of breast is to be done by the opposite hand during self-examination of breast. The person's hand to come down and go up gradually. The breast tissue should not be pinched. After one breast is examined, the other breast would be palpated with the opposite hand in similar manner.

During self-examination of breasts, one must look for:
- Appearance of any lump in breast, armpit
- Any visible changes in size, shape of the breasts, or any changes in appearance of the skin
- Any discharge from the nipple or retraction of the nipple
- Level of the nipples (Fig. 16.3).

If any abnormality is detected, investigations by clinician followed by various imaging techniques are recommended for definite diagnosis of the disease.

Breast Examination by a Clinician

Yearly breast examination by a clinician is also recommended.

Screening by Imaging

Mammography is a low-dose imaging technique, which has reduced the mortality rate. Two types of mammography are in use—film and digital

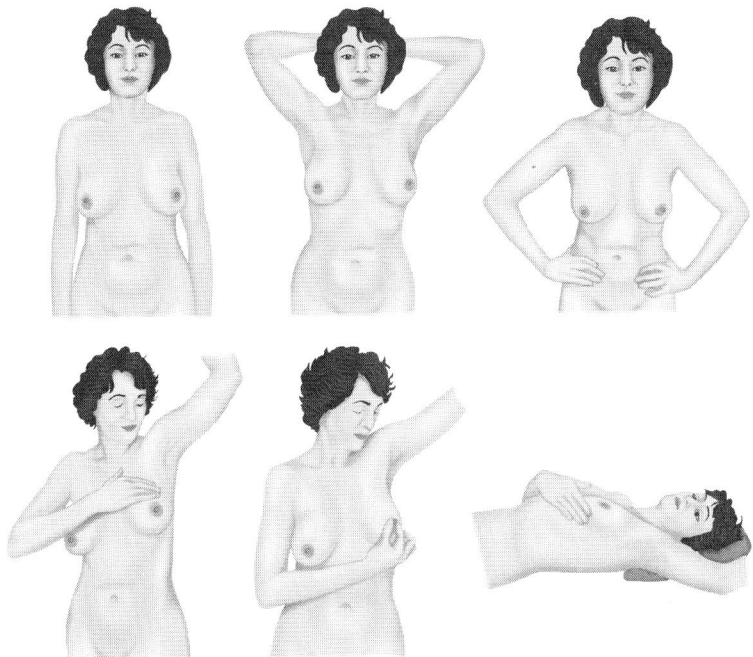

Fig. 16.3: Self-examination of breast.

mammography. Presence of mass, classification, asymmetry, and even abnormal texture are usually detected in mammography. In general, mammography is not that useful in detecting breast cancer in young women aged below 40 years because of the high density of the breast tissue. Below 40 years of age, MRI and ultrasonography (USG) are better modality for detection of breast cancer.

A very recent advancement in mammography is tomosynthesis or 3D mammography, which is able to detect breast cancer in dense breast tissues. This method has been approved by US Food and Drug Administration to use it as routine investigation.

American College of Radiology developed Breast Imaging Reporting and Data System (BI-RADS) for standardization of mammography report. Use of BI-RADS categorization helps in easy diagnosis of breast cancer.

- *BI-RADS 0*: Result is negative
- *BI-RADS 1*: Result is negative
- *BI-RADS 2*: Nodules are benign
- *BI-RADS 3*: Nodules having probability of malignancy less than 2%
- *BI-RADS 4*: Nodules having probability of malignancy between 2 and 94%, biopsy is recommended
- *BI-RADS 5*: Nodules having probability of malignancy 95–100%
- *BI-RADS 6*: Malignancy proved by biopsy.

So, in case of BI-RADS 4 and onwards biopsy is advised.

Positron emission mammography (PEM), breast-specific gamma imaging (BSGI), and molecular breast imaging (MBI) are few modern mammographic techniques currently in use.

Ultrasonography: USG is another imaging technique, which is usually used in follow-up of mammography. It is useful in women of age group below 40 years having high-density breast tissue. This technique is useful in differentiating cysts from masses. Biopsy and other interventions are usually recommended on basis of USG imaging results.

Magnetic resonance imaging: Another imaging-based technique is used to detect malignancies in dense breast tissue and to assess the integrity of silicone implant in breasts. Any previous cancer treatment, changes in hormonal level of the women has impact on the MRI result.

Frequency of Screening

With family history of breast cancer, screening must be started 10 years prior when the relative had the cancer. It can be started even earlier, if necessary. Monthly self-examination, yearly examination by a doctor, and examination by mammography in every 2 years are advised.

OVARIAN CANCER

Ovarian cancer has been named a silent killer because it often lacks any prominent symptoms until the disease has spread beyond the ovary. Symptoms include bloating up sensation, dyspepsia, abdominal pain, difficulty in eating or feeling of heaviness, and mild digestive disturbance. Women between 40 years and 69 years of age who have persistent gastrointestinal symptoms should be investigated for ovarian pathology. Ovarian cancers can be epithelial and nonepithelial. Nonepithelial cancers are found in young patients whereas the epithelial cancers are found in elderly ladies. Ovarian cancer is the most lethal gynecologic malignancy and fourth common cause of death from cancer in the developed world.

Risk Factors

Ovarian cancer risk factors comprise of:
- Family history of ovarian or breast cancer.
- Mutation of *BRCA1* and *BRCA2* gene (mutations in *BRCA1* gene impart 39–46% lifetime risk whereas mutations in *BRCA2* impart 12–20% lifetime risk of developing ovarian cancer). Mutation in *BRCA1* and *BRCA2* usually cause epithelial ovarian cancer. These mutations also can cause breast, fallopian tube, primary peritoneal cancer.

- Mutation in *MLH1*, *MSH2*, *MSH6*, *PMS1*, and *PMS2* cause nonepithelial ovarian cancer. These mutations can also cause colorectal, endometrial, and lower urinary tract cancer.
- Lynch syndrome.
- Early menarche/late menopause.
- Infertility/nulliparity.
- Polycystic ovarian disease.
- Endometriosis.

Statistics and Screening of Ovarian Cancer

According to available data, approximately 22,000 new cases of ovarian cancer and 14,000 deaths related to ovarian cancer are being reported every year from United States. In United States, life time risk of ovarian cancer is 1.2%, which increases to 5% where the first-degree relative has the disease.

In stage I (when the malignancy has not been spread beyond the ovary), ovarian cancer patient has better prognosis, but unfortunately in 70% of the cases the disease is being detected in stage III or stage IV. Only 15% are diagnosed in early stage when the survival rate is 90%.

Hence, screening is necessary in ovarian cancer. Most trials have concentrated on screening asymptomatic women above 50 years of age. Women with no significant family history have 1.3% risk of developing ovarian cancer whereas women with family history of first-degree relative have 3–4% risk of developing ovarian cancer. Women with strong family history of breast and/or ovarian cancer are at life time risk of developing ovarian cancer more than 15%.

Various screening modalities are as follows:
- Pelvic examination
- Transvaginal scan (TVS)
- Doppler
- Tumor markers
- Combination TVS and tumor biomarkers.

Pelvic Examination

Pelvic examination is a part of gynecological evaluation but it is not a reliable method to classify tumors into benign or malignant. It has been calculated that 10,000 routine pelvic examinations would be required to detect one ovarian cancer in population of asymptomatic patients. However, pelvic examination remains the most practical means of detecting early disease. The physician should be suspicious for an early ovarian cancer in any ovary palpable in a patient 3 years or long after menopause.

Ultrasound

Morphology index (MI) based on TVS has been introduced in 1993. There are three parameters—tumor volume, wall structure, and specific volume. Scoring system consists of 0 to 4 in each category with a total screening score ranging from 0 to 12. In 2003, MI was simplified to basic categories—tumor volume, tumor structure. Scoring of both categories ranges from 0 to 5.

Doppler

Arteries formed by neovascularization of malignant tumors are different from normal blood vessels. Absence of tunica media results in reduced resistance. Low resistance indicates neovascularization, which is malignancy.

It is unreliable in predicting malignancy particularly in young patients. In young patients, the low resistance can be due to various infection, pregnancy, and endometriosis. It has no benefit over sonographic tumor MI. By Doppler, malignancy can only be suspected but cannot be confirmed.

Biochemical Markers

Cancer antigen 125 (CA-125) has 50% sensitivity in early stage, but it gives 20–25% false negative test in advanced stage. CA-125 is expressed by 80% of epithelial ovarian cancers, but mucinous cancers, clear cell cancers, and mixed Müllerian tumors often do not produce CA-125. It is also highly expressed in other gynecological and nongynecological conditions also.

OVA-1 Screening Procedure

OVA-1 has been cleared by the Food and Drug Administration (FDA) in 2009 to facilitate clinical decision. This facilitates the referral to an oncologist. OVA-1 incorporates five proteins. Two of them CA-125-II and β-2 macroglobulin are upregulated and three proteins namely transferrin, transthyretin, and apolipoprotein are downregulated. OVA-1 is highly sensitive biomarker for ovarian malignancy. The sensitivity for epithelial ovarian cancer, nonepithelial ovarian cancer, borderline tumors, and metastatic ovarian cancer is 99%, 82%, 75%, and 94%, respectively. When used with standard clinical examination, OVA-1 test predictive value is 93% in premenopausal women, whereas it is 98% in postmenopausal women. However, OVA-1 has not been approved for ovarian cancer screening and surveillance.

Human Epididymis Protein 4

Human epididymis protein 4 (HE-4) detects an antigen derived from *WFDC2* gene that is overexpressed in patients with ovarian cancer. HE-4 is highly sensitive than CA-125 in stage-I ovarian cancer and is expressed more in serous and endometrioid cancer. It has been approved by FDA in June 2008 for clinical use. It aids in monitoring recurrent or progressive disease with epithelial ovarian cancer, but it should be used with other clinical data. It should not be used in monitoring mucinous and germ cell ovarian cancer.

Combination of Ultrasound and Biomarkers

Currently available screening procedure is comprised of measurement of CA-125 glycoprotein antigen, other serological markers and USG or combination of all these methods (known as multimodal screening or MMS). By taking into account all these method, an index score is calculated to predict the risk of ovarian cancer before surgery. This index score is known as Risk Malignancy Index or RMI. It was first proposed by Jacob et al. in 1990. Since then it has been evolved into RMI-II, RMI-III, and RMI-IV. To date only RMI-I and RMI-II have been sufficiently validated.

Calculation of RMI-I:

$$RMI = U \times M \times CA\text{-}125$$

Where,
U = Ultrasound score
M = Menopause status

Ultrasound result is scored one point for each of the following:
- Characteristic multilocular cysts
- Solid areas
- Metastasis
- Ascites
- Bilateral lesion

U = 0 (for ultrasound score 0), U = 1 (for ultrasound score 1), U = 3 (for ultrasound score 2–5).

Menopause status—premenopausal = 1, postmenopausal = 3. Postmenopausal is defined as no period for more than 1 year in a woman of more than 50 years of age or who had hysterectomy.

Cancer antigen 125 is measured in IU/mL and can vary between zero and hundreds or even thousands.

If the calculated index exceeds 200, the patient should be referred to oncologists.

ENDOMETRIAL CANCER

Endometrial cancer is the malignancy of the lining of the uterine wall, which is usually represented with abnormal uterine bleeding (AUB). Hence, it is highly symptomatic. In approximately 90–95% of the cases, the survival is 5 years if the diagnosis is made in the early stage of the disease (when it does not spread beyond uterus).

The AUB can be caused by various reasons and in most of the cases, the reasons are benign. However endometrial evaluation is recommended depending on the bleeding pattern. In postmenopausal women, any kind of bleeding, spotting, or staining is abnormal and must be evaluated by a clinician and by histopathological examination or by endometrial aspiration. In the age group 45 to menopause—frequent bleeding, heavy bleeding, prolonged bleeding, and even amenorrhea for more than 6 months are considered as abnormal and require medical intervention. In women who are less than 45-year-old, persistent AUB in especially fertile, nonobese, or women with Lynch syndrome fall in high-risk group and need further endometrial evaluation.

VULVAR CANCER

Vulva, the female external genitalia, protects the urogenital tract from the foreign bodies. Histologically squamous cell carcinoma is the most common type in vulvar cancer and mostly caused by HPV infection and to some extent by lichen sclerosus. Appearance of vulvar ulcers, plaque, mass, or vulvar pruritus is usual presentation associated with vulvar cancer. Unfortunately, there is no standard method for screening of vulvar cancer.

VAGINAL CANCER

There is annual report of 4,000 new cases and 900 deaths in United States. Features of vaginal cancer are quite similar to vulvar cancer. The most common histological type is squamous cell carcinoma. HPV infection is one of the main reasons of vaginal cancer and most reported HPV subtypes are 16 and 18. Appearance of mass, plaque, or ulcers is considered as presentation of vaginal cancer. No standard method is available for screening of vaginal cancer.

KEY POINTS

Cervical cancer screening is the only screening procedure, which fulfills the World Health Organization (WHO) criteria of screening procedure. Breast and ovarian cancer are detected in the early stage of the disease by screening and unfortunately there are no screening procedures for vulvar and vaginal tubal cancer.

A large number of multidisciplinary research works is going on worldwide for better management of cancer. Despite the enormous efforts, we are still far away reaching our goal, i.e. early diagnosis.
- Screening for gynecological cancer helps to diagnose the disease at earlier stage so that better treatment is possible.
- Cervical cancer can be screened by regular cytological examination as well as by HPV-DNA testing.
- The risk factors for breast cancer include family history of breast cancer, other gynecological cancers and *BRCA1/BRCA2* mutation.

- It is difficult to screen ovarian cancer, as it has no preinvasive disease.
- Usually endometrial cancer is diagnosed early because it presents with symptoms of postmenopausal bleeding or AUB.
- Unfortunately, there are no screening procedures for vulvar, vaginal, and tubal cancer.

SUGGESTED READING

1. Barbara Goff. Early detection of epithelial ovarian cancer: Role of symptom recognition. Uptodate 2017.
2. Joann G Elmore. Screening for breast cancer: Evidence for effectiveness and harms. Uptodate 2017.
3. Joann G Elmore. Screening for breast cancer: Strategies and recommendations. Uptodate 2018.
4. Karen H Lu, Kathleen M Schmeler. Endometrial and ovarian cancer screening and prevention in women with Lynch syndrome (hereditary nonpolyposis colorectal cancer). Uptodate 2016.
5. Karen J Carlson. Screening for ovarian cancer. Uptodate 2018.
6. Lee-may Chen, Jonathan S Berek. Endometrial carcinoma: Clinical features and diagnosis. Uptodate 2016.
7. Lee-may Chen, Jonathan S Berek. Endometrial carcinoma: Epidemiology and risk factors. Uptodate 2017.
8. Sarah Feldman, Annekathryn Goodman, Jeffrey F Peipert. Screening for cervical cancer. Uptodate 2017.
9. Sarah Feldman, Christopher P Crum. Cervical cancer screening tests: Techniques for cervical cytology and human papillomavirus testing. Uptodate 2017.
10. Shambhavi Venkataraman, Priscilla J Slanetz. Breast imaging for cancer screening: Mammography and ultrasonography. Uptodate 2016.

CHAPTER

17

Bleeding after Menopause

Harsha Khullar

Bleeding after menopause is defined as any bleeding per vaginam in menopausal women. It is seen in 4–11% of all gynecological patients. The incidence of bleeding decreases after 3 years after attaining menopause as compared to first 1 year of amenorrhea following menopause (42/1000 vs. 409/1000).

Abnormal bleeding after menopause can be from genital or nongenital sites, which include bladder, urethra, rectum, anus, and lower perineum.

Genital causes include:
- Atrophy
- Polyps
- Endometrial hyperplasia
- Fibroid uterus
- Malignancy
- Postmenopausal hormone therapy.

Nongenital causes include disease in adjacent organs:
- Disease in colon
- Disease in urethra
- Disease in bowel
- Postradiation therapy
- Anticoagulant therapy
- Herbal and dietary supplements.

CAUSES OF BLEEDING

Atrophy

Estrogen deficiency in the postmenopausal female leads to atrophic endometrial surface. There is hardly any fluid in the endometrial cavity to prevent intracavitary friction, which leads to microerosion of the surface epithelium leading to inflammatory reaction. This may result in bleeding or spotting per vaginam (Figs. 17.1A and B).

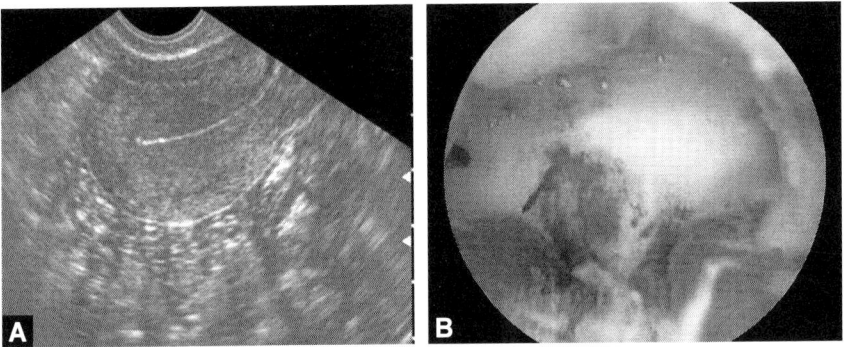

Figs. 17.1A and B: (A) Ultrasonography of vaginal atrophy; (B) Hysteroscopy of vaginal atrophy. *(For Color Version, See Color Plate 3)*

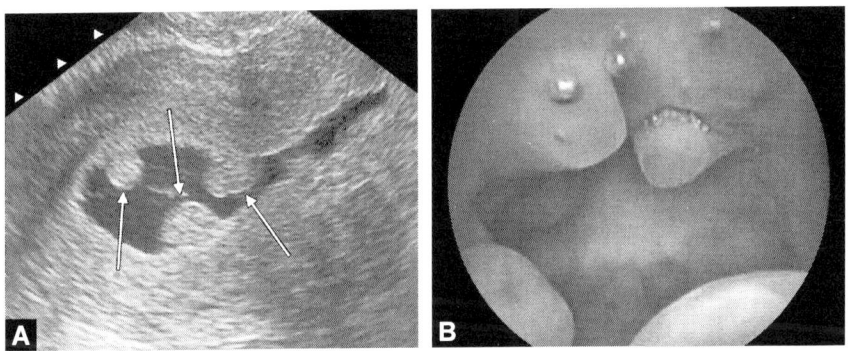

Figs. 17.2A and B: (A) Ultrasonography of uterine polyps; (B) Hysteroscopy of uterine polyps. *(For Color Version, See Color Plate 3)*

Polyps

These are formed due to increased levels of estrogen, which lead to endometrial hyperplasia. These are usually benign endometrial growths and can cause postmenopausal bleeding per vaginam. Treated cases of cancer breast on tamoxifen can have increased endometrial lining due to subendometrial edema (Figs. 17.2A and B).

Endometrial Hyperplasia

Endogenous estrogen production from ovarian, adrenal, and peripheral conversion of fat in obese patients and exogenous hormone therapy may lead to endometrial hyperplasia.

High levels of endogenous estrogen in obese women may be due to conversion of androstenedione to estrone and aromatization of androgen in peripheral tissues to estradiol (Figs. 17.3A and B).

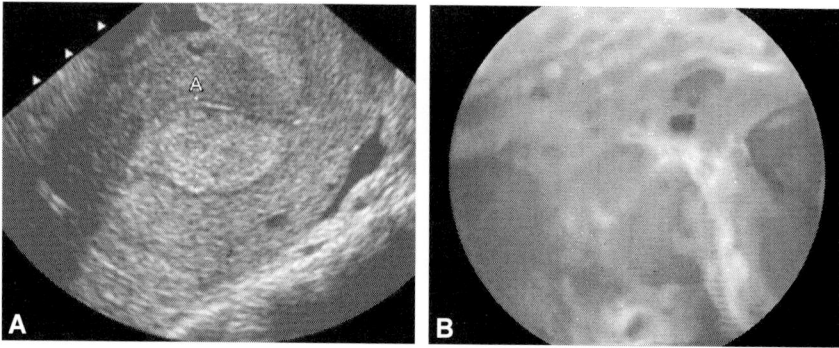

Figs. 17.3A and B: (A) Ultrasonography of hyperplasia; (B) Hysteroscopy of hyperplasia. *(For Color Version, See Color Plate 4)*

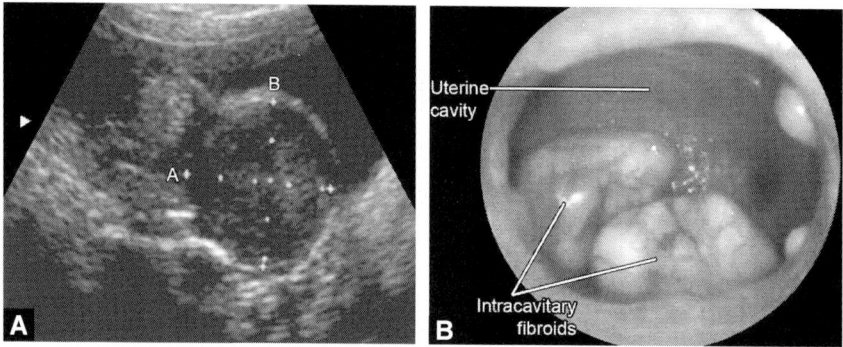

Figs. 17.4A and B: (A) Ultrasonography of fibroid; (B) Hysteroscopy of fibroid. *(For Color Version, See Color Plate 4)*

Fibroid Uterus

The prevalence of fibroids in postmenopausal women is one-tenth of premenopausal women. These rarely can cause postmenopausal bleeding (Figs. 17.4A and B).

Cancer

In 5–10% of women presenting with postmenopausal bleeding, endometrial cancer can be there. The most common genital cancer in women over 45 years of age is adenocarcinoma endometrium.

In 3–5% of uterine tumors, sarcoma of uterus may be there. These may present with postmenopausal bleeding (Fig. 17.5).

Postmenopausal Hormone Therapy

Women taking estrogen therapy may develop vaginal bleeding.

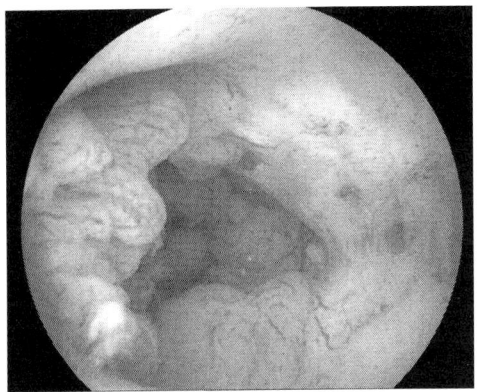

Fig. 17.5: Hysteroscopy of endometrial cancer. *(For Color Version, See Color Plate 4)*

Postradiation Therapy

Due to late effect of radiation therapy, obliterative endarteritis and vascular narrowing of aging and atherosclerosis devascularization of the radiated tissue occur.

Anticoagulant Therapy

It can lead to vaginal bleeding.

Infections

Senile endometritis may present as postmenopausal bleeding. Local infection due to candida can lead to bleeding per vaginam.

Herbal and Dietary Supplements

Supplements rich in phytoestrogens may lead to endometrial hyperplasia and bleeding.

Diseases in Adjacent Organs

Diseases of urethra, bowel, and bladder may cause bleeding per vaginam and may be mistaken as vaginal bleeding.

MANAGEMENT OF PATIENTS WITH POSTMENOPAUSAL BLEEDING

History

- Duration of menopause
- Duration of bleeding per vaginam
- Any precipitating factor like trauma, hormone, anticoagulant therapy
- Contact bleeding
- Changes in bladder and bowel habits

- Family history of breast, ovarian, endometrial, and colon cancer
- History of radiotherapy
- History of diabetes, hypertension, or taking tamoxifen for breast cancer.

A good history may help the clinicians toward one of the major categories of bleeding per vaginam. History of diabetes, obesity, and tamoxifen use in treated case of breast cancer categorize the patients into high risk for endometrial cancer. Complaints of vaginal dryness and soreness with dyspareunia and bleeding after intercourse go in favor of atrophic vaginitis. Patients with history of intrauterine device for contraception use earlier may have forgotten to get it removed and may present as a foreign body leading to bleeding.

High body mass index (BMI) women are at increased risk for endometrial cancer due to increased estrogen due to peripheral conversion of fat.

Examination

- Weight
- Body mass index
- Local examination to see for site of bleeding
- To rule out cervical pathology like polyp and growth
- Systemic examination to rule out hepatosplenomegaly.

Physical examination of external and internal anatomy of female genital tract is important. One should look for suspicious lesions, lacerations, or foreign bodies and to assess the size, contour, and tenderness of the uterus.

Investigations

- Routine
- *Cervical cytology (Pap smear)*: Even if cytology is normal, any visible lesion should be biopsied. Endometrial cells reported in Pap smear in postmenopausal women indicate some endometrial pathology.
- *Ultrasound*: Transvaginal scan (TVS) to see for:
  - Endometrial thickness
  - Echogenicity
  - Adnexa.

The TVS is an acceptable initial test as an alternative to endometrial sampling in postmenopausal women in whom evaluation for uterine pathology, e.g. polyp, leiomyoma, or of the adnexa is indicated.

Diagnostic Evaluation

- *Endometrial sampling*: It is the diagnostic test for women with postmenopausal bleeding. It should be combined with hysteroscopy.
- Hysteroscopy/D and C is the gold standard and any suspicious lesion in the endometrium should be biopsied.

- If benign lesion is discovered, it can be treated.
- Malignant lesions are evaluated and treated according to standard guidelines.

Indications for endometrial biopsy:
- Endometrial thickness is more than 4 mm.
- Diffuse or focal increased echogenicity of endometrium.
- Endometrium is poorly visualized.
- Persistent bleeding.

Management
- Uterine bleeding is usually light and self-limited in postmenopausal women.
- Main objective is to exclude cancer.

Treatment
The treatment will depend on the cause of bleeding.

Atrophy
As hypoestrogenism is the cause, local estrogen cream application is helpful. One must rule out uterine cause before advising estrogen. Breast pathology should also be ruled out.

Polyps
Hysteroscopic evaluation of endometrial cavity and removal of polyps are the treatment of choice. If its histopathology is benign, no further treatment is required. In high-risk patients with history of obesity, diabetes, hypertension, family history of ovarian, uterine or breast malignancy, hysterectomy may be advised if patient is medically fit.

Postmenopausal Hormone Therapy
If patient is on estrogen alone with uterus in situ, she may develop vaginal bleeding. Hormone replacement therapy (HRT) should always be given with estrogen and progesterone in combination. If a woman has undergone hysterectomy, estrogen alone can be prescribed.

In patients with postradiation vaginitis, it might be due to contractures in the vagina. Recurrence of malignancy should be ruled out and local lubricants may be advised.

Herbal and dietary supplement rich in phytoestrogens should be taken with caution as these may lead to endometrial hyperplasia and bleeding.

Local Infection

It should be treated with appropriate antibiotics as against the causative pathogen identified.

Endometrial Hyperplasia

In postmenopausal women, endometrial hyperplasia can be the precursor of malignancy, especially if associated with atypia. Treatment is usually with progestogens and follow-up with serial biopsies. However, careful and regular follow-up of patients at an oncology center is recommended.

Endometrial Cancer

Radical surgery and follow-up according to the stage of the disease are the treatment.

CONCLUSION

- Bleeding per vaginam after menopause is uterine bleeding in menopausal women.
- It is seen in 4–11% of all gynecological patients.
- The incidence decreases with increasing period of menopause.
- Abnormal bleeding after menopause can be from genital or nongynecological sites.
- Endometrial atrophy and endometrial polyps are the most common causes of postmenopausal bleeding.
- In 5–10% cases, endometrial carcinoma may be the cause.
- Primary goal in management of a case of postmenopausal bleeding is to rule out malignancy.
- Pap smear should be the initial test to rule out the cervical pathology and endometrial cells in the Pap smear of postmenopausal women should be considered abnormal and patients need further follow-up.
- The TVS and endometrial biopsy can be used as initial test for evaluating endometrium.
- Hysteroscopy/dilatation and curettage is considered gold standard in evaluating endometrium.
- Management is according to the cause.

SUGGESTED READING

1. Berek and Novak's Gynecology.
2. Williams Gynecology, 15th edition.

CHAPTER 18

Hormone Replacement Therapy in Menopause

Indrani Ganguli

INTRODUCTION

According to The Oxford English Dictionary, replacement therapy is a therapy aimed at making up a deficit of a substance, which is normally present in the body. The loss of estrogen from the body of a woman during the postmenopausal period is a normal physiological phenomenon, so the term HRT should not be used during postmenopausal period. Hormonal deficiency can be replaced only in those women who are congenitally deficient in estrogen or in whom surgery or other treatment have induced premature menopause. Here the term HRT can be used.

Menopause is an important landmark for women. It marks the end of menstruation and the end of reproductive life, and is clearly a biological event.

MYTH OF MENOPAUSE

Robert Wilson, a New York gynecologist com Physician, in 1960s proposed the myth of menopause as an estrogen deficiency disease. According to Wilson, a woman's destiny after menopause without estrogen replacement therapy was to spend the rest of her life as living decay. So, powerful and convincing were his arguments in favor of estrogen replacement that, in the 1970s, estrogen hormone, primarily as estrogen, was one of the top five prescriptions sold in the United States to treat menopausal women. Estimations of hormone use at this time suggested that one-third of women older than 50 years of age were receiving this drug regularly. The beneficial effects of estrogen for the treatment of menopausal women suggested by him were, slowing of ageing process, becoming attractive, decrease in psychological problem, protection of bone and heart disease, prevention of breast and uterine cancer.

The book "Feminine Forever", written by him was sold more than 100,000 copies in 7 months.

ANCIENT INDIA

For over 5,000 years, Ayurveda has acknowledged aging process as a natural phenomenon particularly in menopausal transition. It is not a mistake of Mother Nature that requires hormone therapy. According to the ancient literature, menopause was a balance deficiency. Recommendation was healthy lifestyle with healthy diet and exercises. It was proposed that this should be started early, so that foundation stone is laid down during the reproductive period 20–40 years.

CRISIS OF MENOPAUSAL HORMONE THERAPY

Menopausal hormone therapy faced five crises:
1. First crisis was endometrial cancer published in JAMA. 1946;131:805-8.
2. Second crisis was increase in the risk of breast cancer published in New England Journal of Medicine. 1995;332:1589-93.
3. Third crisis was the Heart and Estrogen/Progesterone Replacement Study (HERS) published in JAMA. 1998;280:605-13. There was no secondary prevention for heart.
4. Fourth crisis [Women's Health Initiative (WHI) study] published in JAMA. 2002;288:872-81.
5. Fifth crisis was Million Women Study published in Lancet. 2003;362: 419-27.

First Crisis

The first crisis was raised by Fremont-Smith et al. with their first case report on the potential relationship between estrogen treatment and endometrial carcinoma. Subsequently, MHT included progesterone along with estrogen either in sequential or in combined continuous formulation. With proper combination of progesterone and estrogen, the risk of endometrial cancer reduces.

Second Crisis

On June 1990, the second crisis occurred with the publication of the Nurse Health Study (NHS). This study indicated that postmenopausal women on a regimen of estrogen only had significantly higher risk of breast cancer than those who never used hormones.

Third Crisis

The third crisis was initiated by The HERS in 1998. It was a randomized trial progestin plus estrogen for secondary prevention of coronary heart disease in postmenopausal women. This study showed that there was no secondary prevention of coronary artery diseases. They concluded MHT might not be the ideal medication for women with established coronary heart disease.

Fourth Crisis

Fourth crisis was the WHI study on July 2002 (WHI study). It was the largest randomized, controlled trial.

WHI Study

It was a randomized control study in which 16,809 healthy and postmenopausal ladies were recruited from 40 centers of USA. In this study, the women were divided into two groups. One group received continuous conjugated equine estrogen 0.625 mg. and medroxyprogesterone acetate (MPA) 2.5 mg while the other group was given placebo. This study reported that 10,000 women who took estrogen and progestin for 1 year might experience seven additional congenital heart disease (CHD) events, eight more strokes, eight more pulmonary emboli, eight more invasive breast cancer, six fewer cases of colorectal cancer, and five fewer hip fractures.

There was increase in coronary diseases and venous thromboembolism (risk increases by twofold). Stroke appeared after 1 year, whereas breast cancer was reported after 4 years.

Fifth Crisis

It was Million Women Study (MWS). The study reported that women who were receiving hormone therapy had more chances of being diagnosed with heart attacks, strokes, venous thromboembolism and breast cancer.

There was further confusion by the publication when the estrogen only arm of the WHI study was terminated because it was confirmed that there was increased risk of stroke after 7 years with an extra eight more strokes per year for every 10,000 women in comparison to placebo. No increase in heart attacks or breast cancer was observed.

Both patients and doctors were confused.

The WHI study and other studies reported since 2002 radically changed the understanding of the risks and benefits associated with MHT—there was a paradigm shift in MHT, prevention was out and symptom relief, if necessary, was the recommendation.

There were various recommendations and consensus reports which came from various societies from USA, UK, and our own menopausal society (IMS). The 16th Progress of Obstetrics and Gynecology, Studd was very critical and vocal of these study results. Some recommendation and conclusions were made and they are as follows:
- Primary indication of MHT is only for moderate and severe menopausal symptoms, vasomotor symptoms, and sleep disruption.
- For each individual, the merits of long-term use need to be assessed at regular interval.

- For vulvar, vaginal dryness, vaginal atrophy, dyspareunia, and atrophic vaginitis, local estrogen is generally recommended.
- Duration of therapy should be shortest and it has to be selective and individualized.
- Doses should be minimum. Prempro approved by Food and Drug Administration (FDA), estrogen 3.5 mg, progestin 1.5 mg (medroxyprogesterone).
- Doses should not be stopped abruptly, it has to be tapered off gradually. It should be gradually tapered off over a period of 3–12 months unless there is a contraindication of using that drug required to urgently discontinue the MHT.
- Women with a uterus should have estrogen–progesterone combination, which can be continuous or combined regimen of cyclical hormone with a minimum of 10 days of progesterone. According to Studd 2014, if breast cancer is due to progesterone then the duration of progesterone should be reduced to 7 days. Progesterone should not be prescribed to women with no uterus.
- Women with a premature menopause should usually be offered MHT till the age of 50 years, which is the average age of menopause. The results from WHI study may not be necessarily applicable to younger postmenopausal women who take suitable doses of various regimens.
- It is important to assess the merits of long-term use for each individual on regular basis. Extended use of estrogen therapy (ET) or estrogen–progesterone therapy (EPT) is acceptable provided the woman is well acquainted with the risks and she should be under strict clinical supervision.
- All women on MHT should have relevant pre-MHT assessment like mammography and ultrasonography (USG) for endometrial thickness, Pap smear and regular annual follow-up tests.
- The decision to continue or discontinue with MHT should be revised at every annual review with a fresh look at the women's needs, preferences, and the medical evidence available at that time.
- The MHT should not be used solely for cardioprotection or cerebroprotection. The effect of MHT on Alzheimer's disease and cardiovascular disease is still uncertain. MHT should not be prescribed only for the prevention of Alzheimer's disease and cardiac disease until some studies prove that it has beneficial effect.

Window of opportunity: It was noted that there was a reduction in coronary events in women aged 50–59 years, who were taking estrogen. This was significant for a complex outcome of myocardial infarction, death, and coronary intervention; but in women aged 70–74 years, there was no beneficial effect. This has led to the implication that there is a "window of opportunity" during the early postmenopausal years for MHT that is beneficial to CHD.

This concept is supported by the findings of Danish studies. In this study, women around the age of menopause were randomized to MHT or placebo for a period of 2-3 years. A follow-up of about 10 years of those women who never had any further treatments showed a significant reduction in atheroma and cardiovascular mortality compared to placebo users.

Present available data show that MHT does not provide protection against stroke; however, it may increase the risk of ischemic stroke.

Women should follow American Heart Association (AHA) guidelines:
- Lifestyle modification
- Exercise
- Proper nutrition
- Weight reduction.

Osteoprotection: There is definitive evidence that EPT is effective in reducing risk of postmenopausal osteoporotic fracture. Because of the potential risks associated with MHT, for women who require drug therapy for osteoporosis, risk reduction alternatives therapy is advised. They are alendronate, raloxifene, and teriparatide, etc.

Recently, a Global Consensus Statement on menopausal hormone therapy clearly suggests that hormone therapy is beneficial and suitable for the prevention of factures related to osteoporosis in women before the age of 60 or within 10 years of the menopause.

Estrogen has another major advantage over bisphosphonates. In the initial 5 years after the menopause, it has been seen that women lose 20% of their skin thickness and collagen. Various studies have shown that estrogens can replace the lost skin collagen and skin thickness.

Recent works on the intervertebral disk is equally promising. The disks are made of collagen and make up one-fourth of the length of the spine. Two different studies performed independently have shown that estrogen protects the spine by maintaining the length of the spine, size of the individual disk, and total disk space. For women below the age of 60 years, estrogen should be the first line of therapy. Bisphosphonates on the other hand should be used in women who have rare contraindication to ET and are nonresponders.

MHT AND UROGYNECOLOGY

Throughout the adult life, the urogenital and lower urinary tracts have shown to be sensitive to estrogen and progesterone. Though Estrogen replacement therapy has been used in the treatment of urogenital atrophy, but its role in postmenopausal urinary incontinence remains controversial.

BREAST CANCER AND MHT

There is much debate about the potential risk between estrogen replacement and breast cancer. A meta-analysis says that women using MHT have higher risk of being diagnosed with breast cancer and it depends on the duration of use. This effect reduces after cessation of MHT largely, if not wholly, disappears after about 5 years and this should be considered in context of the benefits and other risks associated with the use of MHT.

MHT AND OVARIAN CANCER

Global incidence of ovarian cancer is 12.7 per 100,000 at all ages. After diagnosis, only 30% survive for 5 years. Estrogen and progesterone receptors are present on about 60% of ovarian cells. Caution is recommended in prescribing MHT for those women until further studies solve this problem.

It is always advisable to take the lowest effective dose for any medicine as this gives benefits with fewer side effects.

RATIONALITY OF LOW-DOSE MHT

Evidences suggest that for the use of MHT, dose and duration are two important factors for development of any risks. Birth control pill that are now available in the market contains doses of estrogen one-fifth of what it was when they first came out in the market. The women's "HOPE Study" (Health, Osteoporosis, Progestin, and Estrogen), which took place at 57 sites with healthy postmenopausal women, states that low-dose combination of estrogen and progestin is as effective as high doses but with fewer side effects.

HOPE Study

It was a large multicenter, national level study of low-dose MHT trial of 2,805 healthy postmenopausal women. This study was designed to determine the lowest effective dose of estrogen, estrogen-progestin combination therapy for the prevention of bone loss, relief of menopausal symptoms, and endometrial protection.

Benefits of low dose detected were:
- Strong bone
- Decreased number of hot flushes
- Significant improvement of lipid profile
- High-density lipoprotein (HDL) increased 10%
- Bad cholesterol decreased 7%
- Endometrial protection
- Fewer side effects, viz. leg cramps and breast pain.

America Society for Reproductive Medicine (ASRM) have shown that low-dose MHT relieves menopausal symptoms. This has come across as a significant news and a welcome development for the ongoing debate over the risks and benefits of hormone therapy. After years of confusion over its safety, MHT is now being recommended as treatment for the symptoms of menopause.

- Where do we stand now?
- *Is low dose of hormone going to help these ladies?*

Let us review what is happening in the world. All these studies are recent ones.

Osteoporosis

Low-dose Estrogen Patch for Osteoporosis

Menostar-Berlex is a FDA approved low-dose estrogen patch. It prevents osteoporosis without the harmful effects of higher doses. Unlike other estrogen patches, it is not recommended for the treatment of menopausal symptoms like hot flushes, etc.

Effects of Ultra-low Transdermal Estradiol on Bone Mineral Density

In this trial, 417 postmenopausal women between the age of 60 years and 80 years having an intact uterus were randomized to either transdermal estrogen 0.014 mg/day or placebo. Calcium and vitamin D were given to all the patients.

After 2 years, it was noted that the bone mineral density in the lumber spine in the estrogen group raised by 2.6% while 0.6% with placebo. The total hip bone mineral density increased by 0.4% in women administered with estrogen and it decreased by 0.8% in women given placebo. No data is available on fracture risk with low-dose patch.

Cardiovascular

- *Cardiovascular benefits 17β estradiol 1 mg/day*
- *Norethisterone acetate 0.5 mg/day.*

In this study, 100 postmenopausal women were enrolled. There was neither increase in coagulation activation nor any adverse cardiovascular outcome. Low-dose MHT may give cardiovascular benefit.

Low-dose MHT on Menopausal Symptoms, BMD Endometrium, and Cardiovascular System: Review of Randomized Clinical Trials

A literature review of electronic data basis was conducted. Low-dose MHT improved menopausal and vulvovaginal atrophic symptoms, compared to placebo. Less unacceptable side effects included irregular bleeding and breast tenderness. Beneficial effects were seen in bone density.

Sleep

One group was given low-dose conjugated equine estrogens (CEE) 0.3 mg combined with MPA 2.5 mg the next group being CEE—0.3 mg with low-dose micronized natural progesterone 100 mg. Benefit was seen in women who complain of disturbed sleep.

Low-dose intrauterine system releasing 20 µg/24 hours of levonorgestrel (Mirena) with oral E_2 valerate 2 mg (Progynova):
- No clinical or mammography abnormalities were seen.
- Effective endometrial suppression was found.
- Beneficial effects on bone density.
- There was no increase in breast cell proliferation.

Thromboembolism

In this search in the years 1995 to 2005 on venous thromboembolism following results were found:
- In the 1st year of therapy, risks were higher.
- Women using combination of estrogen-progestin had a higher risk of venous thrombosis than those using estrogen alone.
- High-dose estrogen is associated with greater risk of venous thrombosis than low-dose preparations.
- Transdermal use was favorable than oral route.
- Age and overweight where all associated with increased risk.

ESTROGEN REPLACEMENT THERAPY NEWER DEVELOPMENTS

The new science of estrogen action supports the concept that different estrogens acting through the same receptors can induce different biological activities. It has also lead to more research and discovery of new drugs and dosages in order to produce just sufficient levels of hormone to produce adequate results. This has also suggested that the need for estrogen is different for different individuals.
- *Why?*
- *Why does a woman treated with MHT experience so many side effects and a greater risk of cancer?*

All throughout her reproductive years, a woman does not experience such problem with the natural cycle of endogenous estrogens. Mid cycle estrogen can be as high as 150–528 pg/mL. In older postmenopausal women, levels of endogenous plasma estradiol that would otherwise be considered very low in premenopausal women; (<20 pg/mL) are associated with lower risk of hip and vertebral fractures and higher bone density in comparison with undetectable levels when low-dose MHT was given.
- *Is it true?*
- *Is low estrogen a part of the healthy, natural process of postmenopausal phase of life?*
- Is it tailored by the nature in the way our body is meant to function after the childbearing years?

- Is low estrogen good in the sense that it lowers hormone-related cancer risk?

To answer these, we will have to know some relevant points about estrogen in our body. Relation of serum estradiol level and menopausal symptoms, however, is not entirely clear.

- Severity of menopausal symptoms and estradiol level do not correlate. Serum estradiol levels remain at low level although menopausal symptoms instead of persisting, decline beyond 60 years.
- Cases of Turner's syndrome do not have hot flashes, it appears when MHT is started and subsequently withdrawn.
- Some menopausal symptoms are relieved by MHT more than the others. Depression is one which is not significantly relieved by estrogen.

Free estrogen in plasma diffuses into all cells of body freely. Estrogen action depends on the presence of estrogen receptors in cells (ER). There are two estrogen receptors ERα and ERβ. They are located inside the nucleus of the cells. Response to estrogen is dependent on the degree of expression of the receptors.

Estrogen receptor expression can be upregulated and downregulated in body. Regulation of ERα expression is mainly attributed to methylation in tissues. Downregulation by methylation is brought about by an enzyme methyltransferase in DNA. DNA methyltransferase inhibitor (DNAMTi) can be measured. There are methylation inhibitors, which can produce re-expression of ER. Methylation is lowest in ER+/PR+ tumors, intermediate in ER+/PR- tumors and highest in ER-/PR- tumors. Methylation is a mechanism of "gene silencing". ER methylation increases with age.

Does it mean menopause is associated with estrogen deprivation, along with loss of expression of ER in aged? Are they two sides of a coin?

Estrogen Metabolism

Estrogen is metabolized in two ways. Powerful metabolite 16α-hydroxyestrone (16α-OHE1) stimulates target tissues. In breast cancer and lupus, potent metabolites are associated with increased risk and prognosis. Weaker metabolite 2-hydroxyestrone (2OHE1) may slow cell proliferation by binding weakly to cell receptors. The risk of developing conditions associated with estrogen deficiency like depression, heart disease, and osteoporosis may be due to excessive levels of (2OHE1). For optimal health, there should be a proper balance between 2OHE1 and 16α-OHE1.

- 2 (OH) estrone protective or good estrogen?
- 4 (OH) estrone-free radical generator or bad estrogen?
- 16α (OH) estrone genotoxic or bad estrogen?
- 2 (OH) estrone to 16α (OH) estrone ratio is an indicator of cancer risk?

Research is necessary for the following:
- Long-term—duration of low-dose HRT.
- What are the long-term effects?
- Is estrogen level relevant for bad effects?
- Are the receptors responsible for bad effects?
- Is the metabolite of estrogen 2OHE1 and 16α-OH1 ratio important for the bad effects?
- How methylation can help us?

Now, evidence will have to prove that small doses will have the same beneficial effects without any risk. A postmenopausal lady needs to be provided with an endocrine umbrella for at least 20 years beyond 50. The umbrella has to be hole-free (i.e. risk-free).

Can we think of a polypill on the same line as cardiologist use for postmenopausal women, which will relieve vasomotor symptoms, maintain vaginal moisture, induce endometrial bleeding but not producing carcinoma, restore skin collagen, improve breast density but not producing breast carcinoma, prevent osteoporosis, maintain cognitive function of brain, strengthen the sphincters, prevent unnecessary fat deposition. This is far from reality. We will have to depend on other solutions.

For better quality of life and health, menopausal hormone therapy should be accompanied by healthy nutrition and physical and mental exercise as suggested by Ayurveda.

INDIVIDUALIZING MHT

Every woman must be evaluated as an individual. Selective tests must be carried out to establish her healthcare status.

We do not stop playing because we grow old but we grow old because we stop playing.

CONCLUSION

The MHT should be considered as drug, which should be prescribed by an expert who should individualize the dose, route, duration, and drug formulation, according to the needs and desires of the patient.

After full circle of evolution, MHT is back as a drug not as beautifying agent.

SUGGESTED READING

1. Beral V, Million Women Study Collaborators. Breast cancer and hormone-replacement therapy in the Million Women Study. Lancet. 2003;362(9382):419-27.
2. Collins P, Flather M, Lees B, et al. Randomized trial of effects of continuous combined HRT on markers of lipids and coagulation in women with acute coronary syndromes: WHISP Pilot Study. Eur Heart J. 2006;27(17):2046-53.

3. Gambacciani M, Ciaponi M, Cappagli B, et al. Effects of low-dose, continuous combined hormone replacement therapy on sleep in symptomatic postmenopausal women. Maturitas. 2005;50(2):91-7.
4. Lundström E, Söderqvist G, Svane G, et al. Digitized assessment of mammographic breast density in patients who received low-dose intrauterine levonorgestrel in continuous combination with oral estradiol valerate: a pilot study. Fertil Steril. 2006;85(4):989-95.
5. Nelson HD, Humphrey LL, Nygren P, et al. Postmenopausal hormone replacement therapy: scientific review. JAMA. 2002;288(7):872-81.
6. Palacios S, Castelo-Branco C, Cancelo MJ, et al. Low-dose, vaginally administered estrogens may enhance local benefits of systemic therapy in the treatment of urogenital atrophy in postmenopausal women on hormone therapy. Maturitas. 2005;50(2):98-104.
7. Peeyananjarassri K, Baber R. Effects of low-dose hormone therapy on menopausal symptoms, bone mineral density, endometrium, and the cardiovascular system: a review of randomized clinical trials. Climacteric. 2005;8(1):13-23.
8. Shoham Z, Kopernik G. Tools for making correct decisions regarding hormone therapy. part I: background and drugs. Fertil Steril. 2004;81(6):1447-57.
9. Stadel BV, Weiss N. Characteristics of menopausal women: a survey of King and Pierce counties in Washington, 1973-2974. Am J Epidemiol. 1975;102(3):209-16.
10. Wilson R, Wilson T. The fate of the nontreated postmenopausal woman: a plea for the maintenance of adequate estrogen from puberty to the grave. J Am Geriatr Soc. 1963:11:347-62.

CHAPTER 19

Ovarian Cancer

Harsha Khullar

INTRODUCTION

Ovarian cancer is a silent killer as there are no characteristic symptoms. By the time the disease is diagnosed, it is the advanced stage. It can occur at any age and is rightly said that ovaries may stop producing hormones but not the tumors.

INCIDENCE

The incidence of ovarian cancer in different population based registries in India varies from 3.9 per 100,000 to 9.6 per 100,000 women. Ovarian cancer is the second leading cancer of female genital tract.

Epithelial ovarian cancer (EOC) constitutes 85–90% of malignant ovarian tumors of which, various histological types are formed as given in Table 19.1.

The probability for females at birth developing cancer by 85 years of age is one in 81. Approximately 27% of gynecologic cancer is of ovarian origin.

CLASSIFICATION

The staging classification using the International Federation of Gynecology and Obstetrics (FIGO) nomenclature for the carcinoma of the ovary is described in Table 19.2.

Table 19.1: Various histological types of epithelial ovarian cancer.	
Serous cystadenocarcinoma	42%
Mucinous cystadenocarcinoma	12%
Endometroid carcinoma	15%
Undifferentiated carcinoma	17%
Clear cell carcinoma	6%
Undifferentiated, mixed epithelial, unclassified	8%

Table 19.2: Carcinoma of the ovary: Staging classification using the FIGO nomenclature.

FIGO stage	Description
I	Disease limited to ovaries
Ia	Disease limited to one ovary No ascites, capsule intact
Ib	Disease limited to bot ovaries No ascites, capsule intact
Ic	Either stage Ia or stage Ib with ascites containing malignant cells Capsule ruptured
II	Disease involving one or both ovaries with pelvic extension
IIa	Extension or metastasis to the uterus
IIb	Disease spread to other pelvic organs including side wall
IIc	Either stage IIa or IIb with ascites with malignant cells, capsules ruptured
III	Tumor involving one or both ovaries with peritoneal implants outside the pelvis and/or positive retroperitoneal or inguinal nodes
IIIa	Tumor grossly limited to the true pelvis with negative nodes with histologically confirmed microscopic seeding of abdominal peritoneal surfaces
IIIb	Tumor of one or both ovaries; histologically confirmed implants of abdominal peritoneal surfaces, none exceeding 2 cm in diameter; nodes negative
IIIc	Abdominal implants 2 cm in diameter and/or positive retroperitoneal or inguinal nodes
IV	Growth involving one or both ovaries with distant metastasis

(FIGO: International Federation of Gynecology and Obstetrics)

HIGH RISK FACTORS

- Infertility
- Late age at menopause
- Increased dietary fat intake
- Hereditary factors.

The lifetime risk of any women developing ovarian cancer is 1 in 55 (1.8%). Women having first degree relative (mother, sister, and daughter) with ovarian cancer have 4.5 times (8%) lifetime risk of developing same type of cancer. If two or more first degree relatives have ovarian cancer, the risk increases to 55%.

EPITHELIAL OVARIAN TUMOR

The different types of epithelial ovarian tumor are given in Table 19.3.

Table 19.3: Different types of epithelial ovarian tumor.

Serous		
Borderline		
Malignant		
Mucinous		
Borderline		
Malignant		
Pseudomyxoma peritonei		
Endometrioid		
Borderline		
Malignant		
Multifocal		
Clear cell Brenner		
Borderline		
Malignant		
Transitional cell tumors		

Prognostic Variables for Early Stage EOC

Low Risk

- Low grade
- Non-clear cell histologic type
- No ascites
- Intact capsule/without any surface excrescences
- No adhesions.

High Risk

- Clear cell
- Ascitis
- Capsule irregular with growth seen through it
- Dense adhesions.

CURRENT RECOMMENDATIONS FOR WOMEN AT HIGH RISK OF OVARIAN CANCER

- Genetic counseling
- Screening of transvaginal scan (TVS) every 6 months
- Oral contraceptives
- Prophylactic B/L Salpingo-oophorectomy
- In women with family history (F/H) of breast or ovarian cancer mammographic screening after 40 years of age

- In women with F/H of hereditary nonpolyposis colorectal cancer (HNPCC) along with above recommendations, colonoscopy and endometrial biopsy as periodic screening should be done.

MANAGEMENT

Surgical Procedures for Ovarian Cancer

- Surgical staging for presumed localized stage I and II
- Primary optimal debulking surgery for advanced stage III and IV
- Interval debulking after primary chemotherapy in advanced stage disease
- Secondary debulking for recurrent disease
- Second look laparoscopy/laparotomy
- Palliative surgery.

Secondary cytoreductive surgery is done in patients in whom:
- Interval between complete remission and relapse in 12 months or more
- Patients with good response to chemotherapy
- Patients with resectable residual/recurrent disease
- Young patients with high performance status.

Chemotherapy in Epithelial Ovarian Cancer

- Adjuvant chemotherapy for early EOC
- *For advanced stage*: Neoadjuvant (chemotherapy followed by surgery and then chemotherapy)
- *Radiotherapy*: Its value in advanced ovarian cancer is quite limited
- Immunotherapy
- Hormonal therapy.

FOLLOW-UP AFTER TREATMENT

- Second look laparoscopy/laparotomy
- Clinical pelvic examination every 3 months
- CA 125 estimation every 3 months
- Ultrasound every 3 months
- CT/MRI required in patients when CA 125 levels rise during follow-up. This should be followed-up for initial 2 years and then the interval can be increased to 6 months.

NONEPITHELIAL OVARIAN CANCER

- These account for 10% of all ovarian cancer
- These are derived from primordial germ cells of the ovary.

Malignant germ cell neoplasm develop as follows:

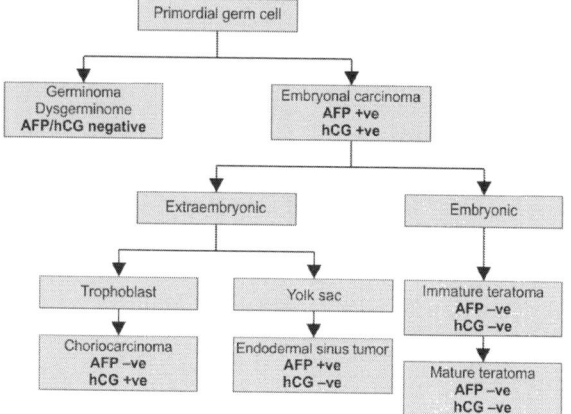

MANAGEMENT OF MALIGNANT GERM CELL NEOPLASM
- Primary surgery
- Chemotherapy for dysgerminoma/nondysgerminoma
- Secondary surgery
- Fertility preserving surgery followed by appropriate chemotherapy should be the mainstay of standard care in young patients.

CONCLUSION
- Ovarian cancer is the second leading cancer of female genital tract
- Late age at menopause, infertility, increased fat intake over the high risk proclaim for ovarian cancer
- The life time risk of any woman developing ovarian cancer is less than 55
- Earlier the diagnosis better is the prognosis
- In younger patient fertility preservation surgery can be done
- Surgical surgery is done for presumed stage I and II
- Adjuvant chemotherapy can be given for early epithelial ovarian cancer.

SUGGESTED READING
1. Berek and Novak's Gynecology.
2. Shaw's Textbook of Gynecology.

CHAPTER 20

Cervical Cancer

Mala Srivastava

EPIDEMIOLOGY OF CANCER CERVIX

Cancer cervix is a disease which can be prevented because it has a long preinvasive stage. Yet in US approximately 12,710 new cases of cancer cervix causing 4,290 deaths were anticipated.

World Health Organization (WHO) states cancer cervix is the most common cancer among women after cancer antigen (CA) breast. About 80% of these cancers occur in developing countries.

Following are the risk factors for cancer cervix:
- Younger age at sexual intercourse
- Multiple sexual partners
- Cigarette smoking
- Race
- More number of children
- Lower socioeconomic status
- Chronic immune suppression
- Infection with human papillomavirus (HPV).

The HPV is the causal agent for cancer cervix, with cofactors as herpes virus and *Chlamydia trachomatis*. HPV is seen in 99% cases of cancer cervix. It is determined as the causative agent in both squamous and adenocarcinoma of the cervix. There are more than 100 types of HPV, of which 14 high-risk types of HPV can cause carcinoma cervix.

MECHANISM OF CARCINOGENS

The HPV causes cancer cervix by interaction of virus protein with tumor suppressor genes.

Symptoms
- Most women are asymptomatic; cancer cervix is identified through the abnormal cytological screening

- Abnormal vaginal bleeding
- Postcoital bleeding
- Postmenopausal bleeding
- In later stages, patients may present with abnormal discharge per vaginum and loss of weight.

LOCAL EXAMINATION

On per speculum examination, cervix could be hypertrophied, firm or suspicious areas could be visualized. There could be a visible growth or the lesion could bleed on touch. The vaginal fornices should be inspected.

Per vaginal and per speculum examination are done, which are particularly conclusive for endocervical cancers. Parametrial extension is identified by nodularity on per-rectal examination.

FEATURES OF CARCINOMA CERVIX ON COLPOSCOPY

- Irregular surface and loss of surface epithelium
- Abnormal blood vessels
- Change in color tone
- Irregular margins.

Adenocarcinoma cervix does not show any characteristic colposcopic appearance. It mostly develops within the endocervix and so, endocervical curettage is needed with colposcopy.

Carcinoma cervix is staged clinically. But imaging modalities like computed tomography (CT) scan and magnetic resonance imaging (MRI) are used to stage the disease. The MRI is more specific and sensitive to CT scan. Hence, MRI is preferred for evaluating tumor size, lymph node metastasis, and for local extension of tumor.

INTERNATIONAL FEDERATION OF GYNECOLOGY AND OBSTETRICS (FIGO) STAGING OF CANCER OF THE CERVIX UTERI (NOVEMBER 2018)

Stage	Description
I	The carcinoma is strictly confined to the cervix (extension to the uterine corpus should be disregarded)
IA	Invasive carcinoma that can be diagnosed only by microscopy, with maximum depth of invasion <5 mm
IA1	Measured stromal invasion <3 mm in depth
IA2	Measured stromal invasion ≥3 mm and <5 mm in depth
IB	Invasive carcinoma with measured deepest invasion ≥5 mm (greater than Stage IA), lesion limited to the cervix uteri

IB1	Invasive carcinoma ≥5 mm depth of stromal invasion, and <2 cm in greatest dimension
IB2	Invasive carcinoma ≥2 cm and <4 cm in greatest dimension
IB3	Invasive carcinoma ≥4 cm in greatest dimension
II	The carcinoma invades beyond the uterus, but has not extended onto the lower third of the vagina or to the pelvic wall
IIA	Involvement limited to the upper two-thirds of the vagina without parametrial involvement
IIA1	Invasive carcinoma <4 cm in greatest dimension
IIA2	Invasive carcinoma ≥4 cm in greatest dimension
IIB	With parametrial involvement but not up to the pelvic wall
III	The carcinoma involves the lower third of the vagina and/or extends to the pelvic wall and/or causes hydronephrosis or nonfunctioning kidney and/or involves pelvic and/or para-aortic lymph nodes
IIIA	The carcinoma involves the lower third of the vagina, with no extension to the pelvic wall
IIIB	Extension to the pelvic wall and/or hydronephrosis or non-functioning kidney (unless known to be due to another cause)
IIIC	Involvement of pelvic and/or para-aortic lymph nodes, irrespective of tumor size and extent (with r and p notations)
IIIC1	Pelvic lymph node metastasis only
IIIC2	Para-aortic lymph node metastasis
IV	The carcinoma has extended beyond the true pelvis or has involved (biopsy proven) the mucosa of the bladder or rectum. (A bullous edema, as such, does not permit a case to be allotted to Stage IV).
IVA	Spread to adjacent pelvic organs
IVB	Spread to distant organs

FIGO STAGING OF CARCINOMA OF THE CERVIX UTERI (2008)

- *Stage I*: The cancer is confined to the cervix
  - *IA*: Cancer not diagnosed by naked eye only. Vertical extension less than or equal to 5 mm and horizontal invasion less than or equal to 7 mm
  - *IA1*: Less than or equal to 3.0 mm in vertical extension and horizontal invasion of less than or equal to 7.0 mm
  - *IA2*: More than 3.0 mm and not more than 5.0 mm vertical extension with an horizontal invasion of not more than 7.0 mm
  - *IB*: The cancer cervix can be seen by naked eye
  - *IB1*: Cancer less than or equal to 4.0 cm in dimension
  - *IB2*: Cancer more than 4.0 cm in dimension

- *Stage II*: Cancer cervix goes beyond the uterus, but not to the pelvic wall or to the lower one-third of the vagina
  - IIA: No parametrial involvement
  - IIA1: Cancer less than or equal to 4.0 cm in dimension
  - IIA2: Cancer more than 4 cm in greatest dimension
  - IIB: There is parametrial extension invasion
- *Stage III*: Cancer goes up to the pelvic wall as well as involves lower one-third of the vagina may cause hydronephrosis
  - IIIA: Cancer up to lower one-third of the vagina, and not reaching up to the lateral pelvic wall
  - IIIB: Reaching up to the lateral to the pelvic wall with or without hydronephrosis.
- *Stage IV*: Cancer goes outside the true pelvis and involves bladder and rectal mucosa
  - IVA: Cancer reaching up to the adjacent organs
  - IVB: Cancer going up to the distant organs.

TYPES OF CANCER CERVIX

Squamous Cell Cancer

Most common is squamous cell carcinoma. Others are:
- Large cell keratinizing
- Large cell nonkeratinizing
- Small cell types
- Less common variants comprise of verrucous carcinoma and papillary (transitional) carcinoma.

Adenocarcinoma

An increasing number of cervical adenocarcinoma is now being diagnosed, especially as the number of cases of invasive squamous cell carcinoma is decreasing. The rise in the incidence of adenocarcinoma has been from 5% earlier to 18.5–27% now.

Adenocarcinoma *in situ* (AIS) is the precursor of invasive adenocarcinoma. Patients with AIS can be treated with conization and they should have close clinical follow-up. Hysterectomy should be considered for patients who have completed their childbearing.

About 80% of cervical adenocarcinomas are predominantly of the endocervical type cells with mucin production, the rest being endometrioid cells, clear cells, intestinal cells, or a mixture of more than one cell type.

Minimal deviation adenocarcinoma (adenoma malignum) is well-differentiated adenocarcinoma.

Villoglandular papillary adenocarcinoma affects young women. They are well-differentiated and have well-defined borders.

Adenosquamous Carcinoma

They comprise of a mixture of malignant glandular and squamous components. It has a poorer prognosis than adenocarcinoma or squamous carcinoma.

Glassy cell carcinoma is poorly differentiated form of adenosquamous carcinoma. Adenoid basal carcinoma and adenoid cystic carcinoma are other variants of adenosquamous carcinoma.

Sarcoma

- Sarcoma of the cervix is also known as embryonal rhabdomyosarcoma, it occurs in children and young adults.
- Leiomyosarcomas and mixed mesodermal tumors involving the cervix and may be primary tumors.
- Cervical adenosarcoma is a low-grade tumor with good prognosis.
- Malignant melanoma may arise de novo. The prognosis depends on the depth of invasion into the cervical stroma.

Neuroendocrine Carcinoma

Neuroendocrine cervical carcinomas are of four histologic types: (1) Small cell, (2) large cell, (3) classical carcinoid, and (4) atypical carcinoid. These tumors are rare.

Patterns of Spread

- Direct invasion into the cervical stroma, corpus, vagina, and parametrium
- Lymphatic metastasis
- Blood-borne metastasis
- Intraperitoneal implantation.

The cervix is commonly involved in cancer of the endometrium and vagina.

Treatment

Radiation therapy can be given in all stages of disease, but surgery is done in Stage I to IIA disease.

Surgery

Sexual dysfunction is less likely with surgery than radiation, because of vaginal shortening, fibrosis, and atrophy of the epithelium with radiation.

MANAGEMENT OF INVASIVE CANCER OF THE CERVIX

Table 20.1 describes management of invasive cancer of the cervix.

Table 20.1: Management of invasive cancer of the cervix.

Stage		Management
Stage IA1	≤3 mm invasion, no LVSI	Conization or type I hysterectomy
	≤3 mm invasion, w/LVSI	Radical trachelectomy or type II radical hysterectomy with pelvic lymphadenectomy
IA2	>3–5 mm invasion	Radical trachelectomy or type II radical hysterectomy with pelvic lymphadenectomy
IB1	>5 mm invasion, <2 cm	Radical trachelectomy or type III radical hysterectomy with pelvic lymphadenectomy
	>5 mm invasion, >2 cm	Type III radical hysterectomy with pelvic lymphadenectomy
IB2		Type III radical hysterectomy with pelvic and para-aortic lymphadenectomy or primary chemoradiation
Stage IIA1		Type III radical hysterectomy with pelvic and para-aortic
IIA2		Lymphadenectomy or primary chemoradiation
IIB		Primary chemoradiation
IIIA, IIIB		
Stage IVA		Primary chemoradiation or primary exenteration
IVB		Primary chemotherapy ± radiation

(LVSI: lymphovascular space invasion)

Simple (Extrafascial) Hysterectomy

Type I hysterectomy is an adequate treatment in stage IA1 carcinoma cervix without lymph-vascular space invasion and not desirous of future fertility.

Radical Trachelectomy

Radical trachelectomy is the surgical management for women with stages 1A2 and IB1 disease who desire uterine preservation and fertility. This can be done vaginally, abdominally, laparoscopically, or robotically, together with pelvic lymphadenectomy and cervical cerclage placement (Table 20.2). This is done ideally for tumors less than 2 cm in diameter and negative lymph nodes.

Radical Hysterectomy

Type III radical hysterectomy includes pelvic lymphadenectomy with removal of most of the uterosacral and cardinal ligaments and the upper one-third of the vagina.

Modified radical or type II hysterectomy described by Wertheim is less extensive. It removes the medial half of the cardinal and uterosacral ligaments.

Table 20.2: Incidence of pelvic and para-aortic lymph node metastasis by stage.

Stage	No of patients	Positive pelvic nodes (%)	Positive para-aortic nodes (%)
IA1 (≤ 3 mm)	179	0.5	0
IA2 (>3–5 mm)	84	4.8	<1
IB	1,926	15.9	2.2
IIA	110	24.5	11
IIB	324	31.4	19
III	125	44.8	30
IVA	23	55	40

Source: Berek and Novak's Gynecology, (2275) Jonathana S Berek, 2012, USA, Lippincott Williams & Wilkins.

Lymphadenectomy

Lymph nodes should be excised and evaluated by frozen section.

Pelvic lymphadenectomy: Patients with bulky cervical tumors and grossly positive pelvic nodes, and when frozen section evaluation is planned, should undergo para-aortic lymph node evaluation to determine the stage of disease and to guide adjuvant therapy.

Para-aortic lymph node evaluation: Enlarged para-aortic lymph nodes are removed. If the lymph nodes are positive for metastatic cancer, then the operation is discontinued and then treated with radiation therapy.

Complications of Radical Hysterectomy

- *Immediate complications*:
    - Blood loss (average, 0.8 L)
    - Ureterovaginal fistula (1–2%)
    - Vesicovaginal fistula (1%)
    - Pulmonary embolus (1–2%)
    - Small bowel obstruction (1%)
    - Febrile morbidity (25–50%)—febrile morbidity is caused by pulmonary infection (10%), pelvic cellulitis (7%), and urinary tract infection (6%). Wound infection, pelvic abscess, and phlebitis occur in less than 5% patients.
- *Delayed complications*:
    - Postoperative bladder dysfunction
    - Lymphocyst formation (<5% patients).
- *Chronic complications*:
    - Bladder hypotonia or, less commonly, atony
    - Ureteral strictures are uncommon.

Nerve-sparing Radical Hysterectomy

It is described in recent years to diminish the bladder dysfunction, sexual dysfunction, and colorectal motility disorders which are commonly seen after traditional radical hysterectomy.

Laparoscopic Radical Hysterectomy

It can be done in highly selected patients.

Sentinel Lymph Node Evaluation

Sentinel lymph node detection has become an important part of the management strategy as a diagnostic tool in carcinoma of the cervix. Thus, a negative sentinel lymph node means omission of lymphadenectomy. Sentinel nodes can be detected in 80-100% of cervical cancer patients, and were confirmed by both laparotomy and laparoscopy. Test sensitivity of 65-87% can be expected with a 90-97% negative predictive value.

Postoperative Management

Prognostic variables for early-stage cervical cancer (IA2–IIA)

Intermediate risk factors for recurrent disease are:
- Large tumor size
- Cervical stromal invasion to the middle or deep one-third
- Lymph-vascular space invasion.

High-risk factors for recurrent disease are:
- Positive or close margins
- Positive lymph nodes
- Microscopic parametrial involvement.

Patients treated with radical hysterectomy who have intermediate or high-risk factors have a 30% and 40% risk, respectively, of recurrence within 3 years.

Lesion Size

Patients with lesions smaller than 2 cm have a survival rate of approximately 90% and patients with lesions larger than 2 cm have a 60% survival rate. When the primary tumor is larger than 4 cm, the survival rate drops to 40%.

Depth of Invasion

When the depth of invasion is less than 1 cm then a 5-year survival rate is approximately 90%, but the survival rate falls to 63-78% if the depth of invasion is more than 1 cm.

Parametrial Spread

Patients with parametrial spread have a 5-year survival rate of 69%, compared with 95% when there is no parametrial spread.

Lymph-Vascular Space Involvement

The reports show a 50–70% 5-year survival rate when lymph-vascular space invasion is present and a 90% 5-year survival rate when the invasion is absent.

Lymph Nodes

The patients with negative nodes have an 85–90% 5-year survival rate, whereas the survival rate with positive nodes ranges from 20 to 74%, depending on the number of nodes involved and the location and size of the metastases.

Primary Radiation Therapy

Radiotherapy can be used to treat all stages of cervical cancer, with cure rates of about 70% for stage I, 60% for stage II, 45% for stage III, and 18% for stage IV.

Comparison of Surgery versus Radiation for Stage IB/IIA Cancer of the Cervix (Table 20.3)

Stage IB lesions less than 2 cm may be treated primarily with an intracavitary source, followed by external therapy to treat the pelvic lymph nodes. The

Table 20.3: Comparison of surgery versus radiation for stage IB/IIA cancer of the cervix.

	Surgery	Radiation
Survival	85%	85%
Serious complications	Urologic fistulas 1–2%	Intestinal and urinary strictures and fistulas 1.4–5.3%
Vagina	Initially shortened, but may lengthen with regular intercourse	Fibrosis and possible stenosis, particularly in postmenopausal patients
Ovaries	Can be conserved	Destroyed
Chronic effects	Bladder atony in 3%	Radiation fibrosis of bowel and bladder in 6–8%
Applicability	Best candidates are younger than 65 years of age, <200 lb, and in good health	All patients are potential candidates
Surgical mortality	1%	1% (from pulmonary embolism during intracavitary therapy)

doses delivered are 7,000–8,000 cGy to point A (defined as 2 cm superior to the external cervical os and 2 cm lateral to the internal uterine canal) and 6,000 cGy to point B (defined as 3 cm lateral to point A), limiting the bladder and rectal dosage to less than 6,000 cGy.

Concurrent Chemoradiation

The use of chemotherapy to sensitize cells to radiation therapy improves local control. The study showed that patients after radical hysterectomy for stage IA2, IB, and IIA disease, chemoradiation is the postoperative treatment of choice.

Chemoradiation is the treatment for stage IIB to IVA disease and that those patients with stage IB2 and IIA disease may benefit from chemoradiation.

A Gynecologic Oncology Group (GOG) study supports the results of previous studies and shows that patients with bulky stage IB and IIA cervical cancer treated with concurrent chemoradiation have survival rates superior to those treated with radiation alone.

Acute Morbidity

Ionizing radiation affects the epithelium of the intestine and bladder and the effect occurs after 2,000–3,000 cGy.

Symptoms may be diarrhea, abdominal cramps, nausea, frequent urination, and rarely bleeding from the bladder or bowel mucosa.

Chronic Morbidity

Radiation-induced vasculitis and fibrosis cause chronic effects. The bowel and bladder fistula rate after pelvic radiation therapy is 1.4–5.3%, respectively. There can be:
- Proctosigmoiditis
- Rectovaginal fistula occur in fewer than 2% of patients
- Small bowel complications
- Chronic urinary tract complications occur in 1–5% of patients and depend on the dose of radiation to the base of the bladder
- Vesicovaginal fistulas are the most common complication.

Chemotherapy for Advanced Disease

Although the combination of cisplatin and topotecan was superior to cisplatin alone, the improvement in overall survival was only 3 months.

Treatment of Cervical Cancer by Stage

Stage IA1 Less than or Equal to 3 mm Invasion

Patients diagnosed with microinvasive cervical adenocarcinoma should have expert pathologic assessment before considering treatment with extrafascial hysterectomy or conization.

Stage IA2 more than 3–5 mm Invasion

Lesions with invasion of greater than 3–5 mm have a 3-8% incidence of pelvic node metastases; thus, pelvic lymphadenectomy is necessary for these lesions. The primary tumor may be treated with a modified radical hysterectomy (type II).

Stages IB1, IB2, and IIA1 Invasive Cancer

Stage IB lesions are subdivided into:
- Stage IB1, i.e. lesions 4 cm or smaller
- Stage IB2, lesions greater than 4 cm.

Stage IIA1 may be managed with either radical trachelectomy or a type III radical hysterectomy, with pelvic lymphadenectomy.

Bulky Stages IB2 and IIA2 Invasive Cancer

Patients with bulky IB2 and IIA2 disease may be treated with either primary chemoradiation or radical surgery. A type III radical hysterectomy with pelvic and para-aortic lymphadenectomy, followed by adjuvant chemoradiation if intermediate or high-risk factors are present.

Stages IIB to IIIB Invasive Cancer

Chemoradiation is the preferred treatment strategy for these patients.

Stages IVA and IVB Cancer

Patients with stage IVB cervical carcinoma are candidates for chemotherapy and palliative pelvic radiation therapy.

Cervical Cancer during Pregnancy

The incidence of invasive cervical cancer associated with pregnancy is 1.2 in 10,000. If the result of the Pap test is positive for malignant cells, and invasive cancer cannot be diagnosed using colposcopy and biopsy, a diagnostic conization procedure may be necessary.

Patients with stages II to IV cervical cancer should be treated with radiotherapy. If the fetus is viable, it is delivered by classic cesarean birth and therapy is begun postoperatively.

Cancer of Cervical Stump

Radical parametrectomy with upper vaginectomy and pelvic lymphadenectomy is the treatment of choice.

Recurrent Cervical Cancer

Treatment of recurrent cervical cancer depends on the mode of primary therapy and the site of recurrence. Patients who were treated initially with surgery should be considered for radiation therapy. Chemotherapy is palliative only and is reserved for patients who are not considered curable by either surgery or radiation therapy.

CONCLUSION

Cancer cervix is a preventable disease. It has a long preinvasive period, well planned.

Primary as well as secondary prevention can go a long way in preventing this disease.

SUGGESTED READING

1. International Collaboration of Epidemiological Studies of Cervical Cancer. Comparison of risk factors for invasive squamous cell carcinoma and adenocarcinoma of the cervix: collaborative reanalysis of individual data on 8,097 women with squamous cell carcinoma and 1,374 women with adenocarcinoma from 12 epidemiological studies. Int J Cancer. 2007;120:885-91.
2. Munger K, Scheffner M, Huibregtse JM, et al. Interactions of HPV E6 and E7 oncoproteins with tumor suppressor gene products. Cancer Surv. 1992;12:197-217.
3. Reimers LL, Anderson WF, Rosenberg PS, et al. Etiologic heterogeneity for cervical carcinoma by histopathologic type, using comparative age-period-cohort models. Cancer Epidemiol Biomarkers Prev. 2009;18:792-800.
4. Siegel R, Ward E, Brawley O, et al. Cancer statistics, 2011. CA Cancer J Clin. 2011; 61:212-36.

CHAPTER 21

Cancer of Endometrium

Mamta Dagar

INTRODUCTION

Endometrium carcinoma is the most common gynecological cancer in developed countries and the second most common after cervical cancer in developing countries. Overall endometrioid carcinoma is the common site and histologic subtype of endometrial carcinoma and of uterine cancer. Endometrioid tumors generally have a better prognosis as they typically present at an early stage with abnormal uterine bleeding where as other histologic types of endometrial cancers (e.g. serous, clear cell, and others) have relatively poor prognosis.

EPIDEMIOLOGY

The lifetime risk of uterine cancer is 2.8%, average age of diagnosis being 62 year. Majority of females with uterine cancer present at an early stage—primary (67%); spread to regional organs and lymph nodes (21%); and distant metastases (8%). Endometrial adenocarcinoma is the most common site and type of uterine cancer.

HISTOPATHOLOGY

Endometrial adenocarcinoma is the most common type of uterine cancer. The two histologic categories of endometrial carcinoma differ in their incidence, estrogen responsiveness, and behavior.

Type I tumor is tumors of endometrioid histology, grade 1 or 2, and comprises about 80% of endometrial carcinomas, has a better prognosis, is estrogen-responsive, and may be preceded by an intraepithelial neoplasm (atypical and/or complex endometrial hyperplasia).

Type II tumors include 10–20% of endometrial carcinomas, grade 3 endometrioid tumors as well as tumors of nonendometrioid histology such as serous, clear cell, mucinous, squamous, transitional cell, mesonephric, and undifferentiated.

RISK FACTORS

The major risk factor for type I (endometrioid) endometrial cancer is relatively an excess of endogenous (obesity) or exogenous estrogen without adequate opposition by a progestin. These women with type I endometrial cancers often have a thickened endometrium on pelvic ultrasound. Other risk factors include tamoxifen therapy, obesity, nulliparity, diabetes mellitus, and hypertension.

Risk factors for type II endometrial carcinomas (serous and clear cell) separately.

Type II endometrial neoplasm is less common, there are fewer epidemiologic data about them than type I carcinomas. They tend to present at an advanced stage. Around 70% of women with uterine serous cancer (USC) and 50% with clear cell cancers present with stage III or IV disease. The average age at diagnosis is older for type II diseases in most studies. Obesity a known risk factor for type I endometrial carcinomas, is not associated with type II cancers. Women with type II tumors are more likely to be parous than nulliparous. Type II tumors have a different racial distribution than type I carcinomas as black women are more likely to be affected than white women.

Diagnosis of endometrial carcinoma is essentially histological based on the results of an endometrial biopsy, endometrial curettage, or hysterectomy specimen.

STAGING AND TREATMENT

Surgery alone is usually curative for low-risk diseases. Women with intermediate or high-risk diseases may benefit from adjuvant therapy.

Staging and Surgical Treatment

Surgical staging of endometrial cancer is in accordance with 2017 Federation of Gynecology and Obstetrics (FIGO) and tumor, node, and metastasis (TNM) classification system (Table 21.1).

Total extrafacial hysterectomy with bilateral salpingo-oophorectomy with pelvic and para-aortic lymph node dissection is the standard surgical treatment for endometrial carcinoma. Cytoreduction is performed when there is evidence of metastasis. Staging may be performed via a minimally invasive route, with robotic assisted laparoscopy, or conventional laparoscopy. Additional routes such as laparotomy or vaginal are often tailored to each patient pathology.

For younger patients diagnosed with endometrial cancer who desire fertility preservation, conservative therapy using progestin (e.g. megestrol acetate or intrauterine progesterone) may be used instead of going directly to

Table 21.1: Primary tumor (T), regional lymph nodes (N) and distant metastasis (M) (surgical—pathologic findings).

Primary tumor (T)

TNM categories	FIGO stages	Definition
TX		Primary tumor cannot be assessed
T0		No evidence of primary tumor
Tis		Carcinoma in situ (preinvasive carcinoma)
T1	I	Tumor confined to corpus uteri
T1a	IA	Tumor limited to endometrium or invades less than one-half of the myometrium
T1b	IB	Tumor invades one-half or more of the myometrium
T2	II	Tumor invades stromal connective tissue of the cervix but does not extend beyond uterus
T3a	IIIA	Tumor involves serosa and/or adnexa (direct extension or metastasis)
T3b	IIIB	Vaginal involvement (direct extension or metastasis) or parametrial involvement
T4	IVA	Tumor invades bladder mucosa and/or bowel mucosa (bullous edema is not sufficient to classify a tumor as T4)

Regional lymph nodes (N)

NX		Regional lymph nodes cannot be assessed
N0		No regional lymph node metastasis
N1	IIIC1	Regional lymph node metastasis to pelvic lymph nodes
N2	IIIC2	Regional lymph node metastasis to para-aortic lymph nodes, with or without positive pelvic lymph nodes

Distant metastasis (M)

M0		No distant metastasis
M1		Distant metastasis (includes metastasis to inguinal lymph nodes intraperitoneal diseases, lung, liver, or bone. It excludes metastasis to para-aortic lymph nodes, vagina, pelvic serosa, or adnexa

(FIGO: Federation of Gynecology and Obstetrics; TNM: tumor, node and metastasis)

surgery. Women deemed to be at low risk of recurrence are considered to be the most appropriate candidates for conservative management.

Patients Stratification

Depending on final pathologic analysis of the uterine specimen and surgical specimen (e.g. lymph nodes or omentum), women can be stratified into risk categories, which aid in decision-making regarding treatment.

Low Risk

Low-risk tumors are grade 1 endometrioid cancers confined to the endometrium, with an excellent prognosis and generally do not require adjuvant treatment.

Intermediate Risk

In the Gynecologic Oncology Group (GOG), intermediate risk is defined as disease that invades the myometrium or demonstrates occult cervical stromal invasion. Other factors used to categorize a higher risk subgroup include the presence of outer one-third myometrial invasion, grade 2 or 3 tumor or evidence of lymphovascular invasion. High intermediate risk is defined as the presence of:
- Three criteria present in a women of any age
- Two criteria present in a women aged 50–69
- One criteria present in a women 70 years or older.

Treatment: These patients often receive adjuvant radiation therapy (RT), although some patients with intermediate high-risk diseases may receive chemotherapy.

High Risk

Women with disease involving the lymph nodes and with uterine serous or clear cell carcinoma of any stage are considered to be at high risk for recurrence.

Treatment: These patients often receive adjuvant chemotherapy, with or without radiotherapy. In most centers, carboplatin and paclitaxel are administered. However, some patients may have received doxorubicin plus cisplatin (with or without paclitaxel).

Follow-up Post-treatment

Post-treatment surveillance is aimed at the early detection of recurrent diseases. Surveillance consists mainly of monitoring for symptoms and physical examination. However, the benefit of surveillance to detect asymptomatic diseases is controversial.

There is no high quality evidence that any specific post-treatment surveillance strategy is associated with improved outcomes. Consensus-based guidelines from the United States National Comprehensive Cancer Network (NCCN) and the Society for Gynecologic Oncologists (SGO) include the following:
- Review of symptoms, physical examination includes per speculum and bimanual pelvic exam every 3–6 months for 2 years, then every 6 months or annually. Frequency of examinations depends upon the risk of persistent or recurrent diseases.

- Genetic counseling for patients with a family history suggestive of lynch syndrome (hereditary nonpolyposis colon cancer).

There is no role of vaginal cytology and vaginal smears in the detection of recurrence compared with physical examination alone. Studies have reported that abnormal vaginal cytology had a sensitivity of 40% and a specificity of 88% in the detection of vaginal recurrence.

In the post-treatment surveillance, the number of computed tomography (CT) scans should be limited as there are concerns about radiation exposure and the risk for second malignancies. Routine use of chest radiography in an asymptomatic survivor is also not suggested.

PATTERN OF RECURRENCE

Commonly endometrial carcinoma recurrences occur 3 years after treatment (68-100%). The sites of recurrence are evenly distributed between vaginal or pelvic and distant (abdominal or lung) metastases. The risk of local recurrence is lower in patients who have received RT and the most common sites of recurrent diseases are vaginal vault, pelvis, abdomen, and lungs.

Studies have indicated that no survival difference between women with asymptomatic versus symptomatic recurrence. Signs and symptoms suggestive of recurrence include vaginal bleeding, abdominal or pelvic pain, persistent cough, or unexplained weight loss.

Asymptomatic recurrences have been detected by the following modalities:
- Physical examination (5-33%)
- Ultrasound abdominal (4-13%)
- Abdominal or pelvic CT (5-21%)
- Chest X-ray (0-14%)
- Cancer antigen (CA) 125 (15%)
- Vaginal vault cytology (0-4%).

Any visible lesion identified during pelvic examination should be confirmed with biopsy as isolated vaginal recurrences are often curable. This has been illustrated in the Postoperative RT for Endometrial Cancer (PORTEC) trial.

Chemotherapy-related Toxicities

The agents used to treat endometrial cancer include carboplatin, paclitaxel, and doxorubicin. All three of these agents may be associated with some toxicities, which persist after treatment such as neurotoxicity and fatigue. Based on the result of GOG 209 trial, carboplatin and paclitaxel are most commonly used adjuvant or first-line treatment.

Pembrolizumab has been approved by the US food and Drug Administration (FDA) for microsatellite instable solid tumor as second-line treatment.

Sexual Dysfunction

Sexual dysfunction may be related to the surgical procedure itself or to adjuvant RT or chemotherapy.

Menopausal Symptoms

The majority of endometrial carcinomas are diagnosed in postmenopausal women but 25% occur in premenopausal women. There are multiple treatments available for menopausal symptoms.

Of available treatments, studies have suggested that progestins are safe and effective for use in endometrial cancer survivors. In addition, nonhormonal options are also safe, including selective serotonin reuptake inhibitors and serotonin or norepinephrine uptake inhibitors, antiepileptics (gabapentin, pregabalin, and clonidine). Other interventions include yoga, hypnosis, relaxation training, acupuncture, and cognitive behavioral therapy (CBT).

- For women with low-risk diseases, estrogen replacement therapy should be administered as first-line therapy which may decrease the risk of long-term health consequences.
- Nonhormonal interventions for menopausal symptoms are suggested for women with intermediate risk or high-risk diseases, if symptoms are not controlled, vaginal rather than systemic estrogen should be prescribed and dosing individualized according to the severity of symptoms and the risk of recurrence.

Lymphedema: It appears to be a significant problem in endometrial cancer survivors, particularly those who have undergone retroperitoneal lymphadenectomy as part of the staging procedure. It most often manifests as lower extremity edema, but might also present as lower extremity heaviness, discomfort, or pain.

Radiation-related Gastrointestinal Toxicity

Adjuvant whole pelvic RT after extensive surgical staging can increase morbidity as it can result in both bladder and bowel dysfunction. Radiation effects can be acute, occurring during, or shortly after completion of treatment or chronic usually beginning 3–12 months following completion of treatment and may last a lifetime. Severe problems are rare, occurring in 4–10% of patient and include rectal bleeding, fistula formation, bowel obstruction, and secondary malignancies. Chronic gastrointestinal (GI) symptoms are more common and include diarrhea, abdominal and rectal pain, bloating, flatulence, and fecal incontinence. External beam RT (EBRT) results in diarrhea scores and bowel symptoms.

FOLLOW-UP CARE

Surveillance should consist of yearly pelvic examinations with visual examination of the vaginal mucosa and vaginal cuff via speculum examination and digital rectovaginal examination. Symptoms such as vaginal bleeding or postcoital bleeding, pelvic pressure, or change in bowel or bladder habits should be carefully investigated to rule out recurrent diseases.

Patients younger than 50 with endometrial cancer may be at increased risk for colon cancer [hereditary nonpolyposis colorectal cancer (HNPCC) or lynch syndrome] and microsatellite instability testing should be performed on the patient's endometrial cancer tissue as a screening test.

Staging and Surgical Treatment of Endometrial Cancer

Adjuvant Therapy

Decision about adjuvant treatment for endometrial carcinoma is based on clinicopathologic factors (e.g. grade, tumor size, and patient's age). Other factors may also impact adjuvant treatment decision such as lower uterine segment involvement and positive peritoneal cytology.

Fertility Preservation

Women who are at low-risk endometrial cancer willing to preserve fertility may be treated with progestin therapy (e.g. megestrol acetate). A complete evaluation prior to commencing medical therapy by endometrial sampling and imaging is required to confirm that the tumor is confined to the uterus and is grade 1 or 2.

PROGNOSIS

Stage, grade, and histological subtyping are important prognosis factors of endometrial carcinoma.

Majority of women with endometrial carcinoma have a good, as the most of them have endometrioid histology and present at an early stage of diseases.

The 5-year survival rate for stage I diseases is around 80–90%, for stage II is 70–80%, and for stage III and IV is 20–60%.

CONCLUSION

- Endometrium carcinoma is the most common gynecological cancer after cervical cancer in developing countries.
- Endometrial adenocarcinoma is the most common type of uterine cancer. The two histologic categories of endometrial carcinoma differ in their incidence, estrogen responsiveness, and behavior.

- Diagnosis of endometrial carcinoma is essentially histological based on the results of an endometrial biopsy, endometrial curettage, or hysterectomy specimen.
- Surgery alone is usually curative for low-risk diseases. Women with intermediate or high-risk diseases may benefit from adjuvant therapy.
- Stage, grade and histological subtyping are important prognosis factors of endometrial carcinoma.
- Decision about adjuvant treatment for endometrial carcinoma is based on clinicopathologic factors (e.g. grade, tumor size, and patient's age).

SUGGESTED READING

1. Andreyev HJ. Gastrointestinal problems after pelvic radiotherapy: the past, the present and the future. Clin Oncol (R Coll Radiol). 2007;19:790-9.
2. Ben Arie A, Lavie O, Gdalevich M, et al. Temporal pattern of recurrence of stage I endometrial cancer in relation to histological risk factors. Eur J Surg Oncol. 2012;38:166-9.
3. Bruegl AS, Djordjevic B, Urbauer DL, et al. Utility of MLH1 methylation analysis in the clinical evaluation of Lynch syndrome in women with endometrial cancer. Curr Pharm Des. 2014;20:1655-63.
4. Felix AS, Weissfeld JL, Stone RA, et al. Factors associated with type I and type II endometrial cancer. Cancer Causes Control. 2010;21:1851-6.
5. Fung-Kee-Fung M, Dodge J, Elit L, et al. Follow-up after primary therapy for endometrial cancer: a systematic review. Gynecol Oncol. 2006;101:520-9.
6. Hitchcock CL, Prior JC. Oral micronized progesterone for vasomotor symptoms—a placebo-controlled randomized trial in healthy postmenopausal women. Menopause. 2012;19:886-93.
7. Hunter MS, Grunfeld EA, Mittal S, et al. Menopausal symptoms in women with breast cancer: prevalence and treatment preferences. Psychooncology. 2004;13:769-78.
8. Lewin SN, Herzog TJ, Barrena Medel NI, et al. Comparative Performance of the 2009 International Federation of Gynecology and Obstetrics' Staging System for Uterine Corpus Cancer. Obstet Gynecol. 2010;116:1141-9.
9. Loprinzi CL, Sloan J, Stearns V, et al. Newer antidepressants and gabapentin for hot flashes: an individual patient pooled analysis. J Clin Oncol. 2009;27:2831-7.
10. Miller DS, Filiaci G, Mannel R, et al. Randomized Phase III Noninferiority Trial of First Line Chemotherapy for Metastatic or Recurrent Endometrial Carcinoma: A Gynecologic Oncology Group Study. LBA2. Presented at the 2012. Austin TX: Society of Gynecologic Oncology Annual Meeting; 2012.
11. Moore KN, Fader AN. Uterine papillary serous carcinoma. Clin Obstet Gynecol. 2011;54:278-91.
12. National Cancer Institute. Cancer Stat Facts: Uterine Cancer. [online] Available from: http://seer.cancer.gov/statfacts/html/corp.html [Accessed December, 2016].
13. National Comprehensive Cancer Network (NCCN). NCCN Clinical practice guidelines in oncology. [online] Available from: https://www.nccn.org/professionals/physician_gls/pdf/neuroendocrine.pdf [Accessed December,2018].
14. Nout RA, Putter H, Jürgenliemk-Schulz IM, et al. Quality of life after pelvic radiotherapy or vaginal brachytherapy for endometrial cancer: first results of the randomized PORTEC-2 trial. J Clin Oncol. 2009;27:3547-56.

15. Novetsky AP, Kuroki LM, Massad LS, et al. The utility and management of vaginal cytology after treatment for endometrial cancer. Obstet Gynecol. 2013;121:129-35.
16. Otsuka I, Uno M, Wakabayashi A, et al. Predictive factors for prolonged survival in recurrent endometrial carcinoma: Implications for follow-up protocol. Gynecol Oncol. 2010;119:506-10.
17. Ott PA, Bang YJ, Berton-Rigaud D, et al. Safety and Antitumor Activity of Pembrolizumab in Advanced Programmed Death Ligand 1-Positive Endometrial Cancer: Results From the KEYNOTE-028 Study. J Clin Oncol. 2017;35:2535-41.
18. Thomas M, Mariani A, Wright JD, et al. Surgical management and adjuvant therapy for patients with uterine clear cell carcinoma: a multi-institutional review. Gynecol Oncol. 2008;108:2937.
19. Torre LA, Bray F, Siegel RL, et al. Global cancer statistics, 2012. CA Cancer J Clin. 2015; 65:87-108.
20. Wright JD, Fiorelli J, Schiff PB, et al. Racial disparities for uterine corpus tumors: changes in clinical characteristics and treatment over time. Cancer. 2009;115: 1276-85.

CHAPTER 22

Management of Breast Cancer: An Overview

Rakesh Kumar Koul

INTRODUCTION

Breast cancer has been the most frequent cause of life-threatening cancer in females and a leading cause of cancer-related mortality in underdeveloped and developing countries. In the later decades of last century there was worldwide surge in the incidence of breast cancers. It was mainly attributed to the widespread use of screening mammography. Besides this, other factors like change in reproductive pattern and change in lifestyles in relation to the diet, physical activity, and use of oral hormonal contraceptive were important contributing factors.

SYMPTOMS

Breast malignancies are detected either on screening mammogram or following the evaluation of any of the following symptoms:
- Lump in breast and/or axilla.
- Change in shape and size of breast.
- Skin changes including dimpling, ulceration or widespread redness.
- Nipple retraction.
- Nipple discharge, especially if it is blood-stained.

EVALUATION OF BREAST MALIGNANCY

Evaluation of breast cancer by *"triple assessment"* includes the following described here.

Clinical Examination

It includes:
- *Clinical breast examination*: This is undertaken by the clinician as a part of evaluation of signs and symptoms confined to breast or as an adjunct to breast cancer screening program. In the later case it is undertaken on

annual basis, starting at 40 years of age in a female with mild to moderate risk of breast malignancy.
- *Breast self examination*: It is undertaken by the individual on self at every 3-month intervals.

Imaging

It includes:
- *Diagnostic mammogram*: It is usually done in two views—craniocaudal (CC) and mediolateral oblique (MLO). It determines the shape, size and location of the breast abnormality as well as the status of the axillary lymph nodes.
- *Sonomammogram*: It is usually used in conjunction with mammogram. It provides valuable information regarding the nature of the breast lumps and can differentiate between cystic breast lumps from the solid ones.
- *Magnetic resonance imaging (MRI)*: MR mammogram has a role in characterizing an indeterminate breast lesion, detecting occult carcinoma in case of metastasis of unknown origin to axillary lymph nodes, evaluation of multifocal and bilateral breast tumors, evaluation of invasive lobular carcinoma, and recurrent breast malignancies.
- *Positron emission tomography (PET) scan*: PET scan is utilized for clinical staging of locally advanced breast malignancies, including inflammatory breast cancer (IBC). It is also used for assessing the response of breast cancer to neoadjuvant chemotherapy.

Needle Biopsy

Image-guided core needle biopsies of the breast masses is preferable to fine-needle aspiration cytology (FNAC) or excision biopsy as most of the times it provides accurate diagnosis without the distortion of breast architecture thus minimizing the chances of unwanted surgical interventions. Also, core biopsy tissue can be subjected to immunohistochemical investigations for further characterization of breast tumors.

HISTOLOGY

The common varieties of breast malignancies are as follows:
- The most common type of breast malignancy is infiltrating ductal carcinoma and it constitutes 75% of breast cancers.
- Infiltrating lobular carcinoma comprises approximately 15% of invasive breast cancers.
- Medullary carcinoma is seen in about 5% of cases.
- Mucinous carcinoma also accounts of 5% of invasive breast cancers.
- Other rare breast cancers include tubular carcinoma, papillary carcinoma, metaplastic breast cancer, and Paget disease.

All of the following histological features are important in deciding on a course of treatment for any breast tumor:
- Size
- Status of surgical margin
- Presence or absence of estrogen receptor (ER) and progesterone receptor (PR)
- Nuclear and histologic grade
- Proliferation
- Vascular invasion
- Tumor necrosis
- Quantity of intraductal component
- Human epidermal growth factor (HER2) status.

HER2 Testing

Breast cancer specimens should initially undergo HER2 testing by a validated immunohistochemistry (IHC) assay.

The scoring method for HER2 expression is based on the cell membrane staining pattern and is as follows:
- 3+: Positive for HER2 protein expression
- 2+: Equivocal for HER2 protein expression. Equivocal IHC results can be seen in 15% of invasive breast cancers
- 1+: Negative is considered when there is weak or incomplete membrane staining in any tumor cells
- 0: Negative for HER2 protein expression; no staining.

Breast cancer specimens with equivocal IHC results undergo validation with a *HER2* gene amplification method, such as fluorescence in situ hybridization (FISH) for confirmation of results. The interpretation for HER2 FISH testing [ratio of HER2 to chromosome 17 centromere (HER2/CEP17) and gene copy number] is as follows:
- *Positive HER2 amplification*: HER2:CEP17 ratio is greater than 2.2 or *HER2* gene copy is greater than 6.0
- Equivocal *HER2* amplification: HER2:CEP17 ratio of 1.8–2.2 or *HER2* gene copy of 4.0–6.0
- Negative *HER2* amplification: HER2:CEP17 ratio is less than 1.8 or *HER2* gene copy of less than 4.0.

FURTHER CLINICAL STAGING

After confirmation of the diagnosis of breast malignancy and its IHC status, further clinical staging is required. National Comprehensive Cancer Network (NCCN) 2017 guidelines recommend the following additional investigations.

Early Stage Breast Malignancy (up to Stage IIB)
- Complete blood count (CBC)
- Liver function test, including alkaline phosphatase
- Bone scan, in patients with localized bone pain or raised alkaline phosphatase levels
- Contrast-enhanced computed tomography (CT) or contrast-enhanced MRI of whole abdomen in patients with abnormal liver function tests, abdominal symptoms, or abnormal physical examination of the abdomen or pelvis
- Contrast-enhanced CT of chest in patients with pulmonary symptoms.

Locally Advanced/Metastatic Breast Cancer (Stage IIIA or More)
Investigations needed to be conducted are:
- CBC
- LFT including alkaline phosphatase
- Whole body bone scan
- Contrast-enhanced CT or contrast-enhanced MRI of whole abdomen
- Contrast-enhanced CT of chest
- PET-CT (optional), instead of bone scan, CT abdomen and CT chest.

BREAST CANCER STAGING
American Joint Committee on Cancer (AJCC) groups breast cancer into four stages, based on TNM (Tumor, Node, and Metastasis). The latest 8th edition of AJCC however inserts following changes into the staging system:
- The IHC tumor markers are incorporated to redefine and refine the prognosis.
- Lobular carcinoma in situ (LCIS) has been eliminated from the staging system as it is now considered a risk factor only and not a malignancy.
- Genomic assays are now used to downstage ER-positive and lymph node-negative tumors.

TNM Classification for Breast Cancer

Primary Tumor (T)

TX	:	Primary tumor cannot be assessed
T0	:	No evidence of primary tumor
Tis	:	Carcinoma in situ
Tis (DCIS)	:	Ductal carcinoma in situ
Tis (LCIS)	:	Lobular carcinoma in situ
Tis (Paget)	:	Paget disease of the nipple NOT associated with invasive carcinoma and/or carcinoma in situ (DCIS and/or LCIS) in

the underlying breast parenchyma. Carcinomas in the breast parenchyma associated with Paget disease are categorized based on the size and characteristics of the parenchymal disease, although the presence of Paget disease should still be noted.

T1	:	Tumor ≤20 mm in greatest dimension
T1mi	:	Tumor ≤1 mm in greatest dimension
T1a	:	Tumor >1 mm but ≤5 mm in greatest dimension
T1b	:	Tumor >5 mm but ≤10 mm in greatest dimension
T1c	:	Tumor >10 mm but ≤20 mm in greatest dimension
T2	:	Tumor >20 mm but ≤50 mm in greatest dimension
T3	:	Tumor >50 mm in greatest dimension
T4	:	Tumor of any size with direct extension to the chest wall and/or to the skin (ulceration or skin nodules)
T4a	:	Extension to chest wall, not including only pectoralis muscle adherence or invasion
T4b	:	Ulceration and/or ipsilateral satellite nodules and/or edema (including peau d'orange) of the skin, which do not meet the criteria for inflammatory carcinoma
T4c	:	Both T4a and T4b
T4d	:	Inflammatory carcinoma

Regional Lymph Nodes (N)

Clinical:

NX	:	Regional lymph nodes cannot be assessed (e.g. previously removed)
N0	:	No regional lymph node metastasis
N1	:	Metastasis to movable ipsilateral level I, II axillary lymph node(s)
N2	:	Metastases in ipsilateral level I, II axillary lymph nodes that are clinically fixed or matted or in clinically detected* ipsilateral internal mammary nodes in the *absence* of clinically evident axillary lymph node metastasis
N2a	:	Metastases in ipsilateral level I, II axillary lymph nodes fixed to one another (matted) or to other structures
N2b	:	Metastases only in clinically detected* ipsilateral internal mammary nodes and in the *absence* of clinically evident level I, II axillary lymph node metastases
N3	:	Metastases in ipsilateral infraclavicular (level III axillary) lymph node(s), with or without level I, II axillary node involvement, or in clinically detected* ipsilateral internal

---

*"Clinically detected" is defined as detected by imaging studies (excluding lymphoscintigraphy) or by clinical examination and having characteristics highly suspicious for malignancy or a presumed pathologic macrometastasis on the basis of FNA biopsy with cytologic examination.

		mammary lymph node(s) and in the *presence* of clinically evident level I, II axillary lymph node metastasis; or metastasis in ipsilateral supraclavicular lymph node(s), with or without axillary or internal mammary lymph node involvement
N3a	:	Metastasis in ipsilateral infraclavicular lymph node(s)
N3b	:	Metastasis in ipsilateral internal mammary lymph node(s) and axillary lymph node(s)
N3c	:	Metastasis in ipsilateral supraclavicular lymph node(s)

Pathologic (pN):

pNX	:	Regional lymph nodes cannot be assessed (for example, previously removed, or not removed for pathologic study)
pN0	:	No regional lymph node metastasis identified histologically. *Note*: Isolated tumor cell clusters (ITCs) are defined as small clusters of cells ≤0.2 mm, or single tumor cells, or a cluster of <200 cells in a single histologic cross-section; ITCs may be detected by routine histology or by immunohistochemical (IHC) methods; nodes containing only ITCs are excluded from the total positive node count for purposes of N classification but should be included in the total number of nodes evaluated
pN0 (i-)	:	No regional lymph node metastases histologically, negative IHC
pN0 (i+)	:	Malignant cells in regional lymph node(s) ≤0.2 mm [detected by hematoxylin and eosin (H&E) stain or IHC, including ITC]
pN0 (mol-)	:	No regional lymph node metastases histologically, negative molecular findings [reverse transcriptase polymerase chain reaction [RT-PCR])
pN0 (mol+)	:	Positive molecular findings (RT-PCR) but no regional lymph node metastases detected by histology or IHC
pN1	:	Micrometastases; or metastases in 1-3 axillary lymph nodes and/or in internal mammary nodes, with metastases detected by sentinel lymph node biopsy but not clinically detected⁺
pN1mi	:	Micrometastases (>0.2 mm and/or >200 cells, but none >2.0 mm)
pN1a	:	Metastases in 1-3 axillary lymph nodes (at least 1 metastasis >2.0 mm)
pN1b	:	Metastases in internal mammary nodes, with micrometastases or macrometastases detected by sentinel lymph node biopsy but not clinically detected⁺
pN1c	:	Metastases in 1-3 axillary lymph nodes and in internal mammary lymph nodes, with micrometastases or macrometastases detected by sentinel lymph node biopsy but not clinically detected⁺

pN2	:	Metastases in 4-9 axillary lymph nodes or in clinically detected⁺ internal mammary lymph nodes in the absence of axillary lymph node metastases
pN2a	:	Metastases in 4-9 axillary lymph nodes (at least 1 tumor deposit >2.0 mm)
pN2b	:	Metastases in clinically detected⁺ internal mammary lymph nodes in the absence of axillary lymph node metastases
pN3	:	Metastases in ≥10 axillary lymph nodes; or in infraclavicular (level III axillary) lymph nodes; or in clinically detected⁺ ipsilateral internal mammary lymph nodes in the presence of ≥1 positive level I, II axillary lymph nodes; or in >3 axillary lymph nodes and in internal mammary lymph nodes, with micrometastases or macrometastases detected by sentinel lymph node biopsy but not clinically detected⁺; or in ipsilateral supraclavicular lymph nodes
pN3a	:	Metastases in ≥10 axillary lymph nodes (at least 1 tumor deposit >2.0 mm); or metastases to the infraclavicular (level III axillary lymph) nodes
pN3b	:	Metastases in clinically detected⁺ ipsilateral internal mammary lymph nodes in the presence of ≥1 positive axillary lymph nodes; or in >3 axillary lymph nodes and in internal mammary lymph nodes, with micrometastases or macrometastases detected by sentinel lymph node biopsy but not clinically detected⁺
pN3c	:	Metastases in ipsilateral supraclavicular lymphnodes

Distant Metastasis (M)

M0	:	No clinical or radiographic evidence of distant metastasis
cM0(i+)	:	No clinical or radiographic evidence of distant metastases, but deposits of molecularly or microscopically detected tumor cells in circulating blood, bone marrow, or other nonregional nodal tissue that are no larger than 0.2 mm in a patient without symptoms or signs of metastases
M1	:	Distant detectable metastases as determined by classic clinical and radiographic means and/or histologically proven >0.2 mm

Histologic Grade (G)

GX	:	Grade cannot be assessed
G1	:	Low combined histologic grade (favorable)
G2	:	Intermediate combined histologic grade (moderately favorable)
G3	:	High combined histologic grade (unfavorable)

⁺"Clinically detected" is defined as detected by imaging studies (except lymphoscintigraphy) or by clinical examination and having characteristics highly suspicious for malignancy or a presumed pathologic macrometastasis on the basis of FNA biopsy with cytologic examination.

Source: [Guideline] NCCN Clinical Practice Guidelines in Oncology: Breast Cancer. V 1.2016. National Comprehensive Cancer Network. Available at http://www.nccn.org/professionals/physician_gls/pdf/breast.pdf. Version 3.2018 — October 25, 2018; Accessed: December 7, 2018.

Stage Grouping

Stage	T	N	M
0	Tis	N0	M0
IA	T1	N0	M0
IB	T0	N1mi	M0
	T1	N1mi	M0
IIA	T0	N1	M0
	T1	N1	M0
	T2	N0	M0
IIB	T2	N1	M0
	T3	N0	M0
IIIA	T0	N2	M0
	T1	N2	M0
	T2	N2	M0
	T3	N1	M0
	T3	N2	M0
IIIB	T4	N0	M
	T4	N1	M0
	T4	N2	M0
IIIC	Any T	N3	M0
IV	Any T	Any N	M1

MOLECULAR PROFILING ASSAYS

Onco type Dx Assay

A. The "Onco *type* Dx" assay is reserved for women with early-stage ER-positive, node-negative breast cancer treated with tamoxifen, where the recurrence score (RS) correlates with both relapse-free interval and overall survival (OS). This is a RT-PCR based assay of 21 genes (16 cancer genes and 5 reference genes), performed on paraffin-embedded breast tumor tissue.

By using a formula based on the expression of these genes, an RS can be calculated that correlates with the likelihood of distant recurrence at 10 years. Breast tumor RS and risk levels are as follows:
- Below 18, low risk
- 18–30, intermediate risk
- Above 30, high risk.

Onco *type* Dx assay can predict benefit from chemotherapy and hormonal therapy in hormone-sensitive, node-negative tumors as shown by the National Surgical Adjuvant Breast and Bowel Project (NSABP) B-14 and B-20 studies.

Women with a low RS showed a significantly greater improvement in disease-free survival (DFS) with the addition of tamoxifen; no additional benefit was derived from the addition of chemotherapy. In contrast, women with a high RS had a significant improvement in DFS with the addition of chemotherapy to hormonal therapy (tamoxifen).

MammaPrint Assay

The *MammaPrint* assay is a genetic test that measures the activity of 70 genes to determine the 5- to 10-year relapse risk for women diagnosed with early breast cancer. MammaPrint test results are reported as either a low-risk or a high-risk RS:
- A low-risk score means that the cancer has a 10% risk of coming back within 10 years without any additional treatments after surgery.
- A high-risk score means that the cancer has a 29% risk of coming back within 10 years without any additional treatments after surgery.

MANAGEMENT OF PREINVASIVE BREAST TUMORS (STAGE 0)

Ductal Carcinoma In Situ (DCIS)

The goal of treatment of ductal carcinoma in situ (DCIS) is prevention of its progression to invasive cancer. Modes of its treatment are surgery (lumpectomy or mastectomy), radiotherapy, and endocrine therapy. NCCN recommends breast conservation surgery (BCS) followed by adjuvant external-beam radiotherapy (EBRT), or total mastectomy with or without sentinel lymph nodal biopsy (SLNB). Complete resection should be ensured by margin status and postexcision mammography. EBRT, post BCS decreased incidence of recurrences by 60%, half of which are approximately invasive cancers. In ER-positive patients of DCIS, NCCN recommends treatment with tamoxifen (in premenopausal and postmenopausal) or anastrozole (in postmenopausal especially if they are <60 years of age) for 10 years.

Lobular Carcinoma In Situ (LCIS)

Treatment of LCIS is controversial. 17–27% of LCIS diagnosed on core needle biopsy alone are upstaged to invasive ductal cancers or DCIS after larger surgical excision. Also more than 4 foci of LCIS on single core may also have the risk of upstaging on surgical biopsy. NCCN recommends that LCIS of usual (classical) type having less than 4 foci of LCIS on a single core of biopsy without associated imaging distortion other than calcification will require follow up which includes interval history and clinical examination every 6–12 months and annual mammogram. Pleomorphic LCIS or LCIS with necrosis carries higher risk of getting upstaged and is advised resection.

TREATMENT OF EARLY STAGE INVASIVE BREAST CANCER

Invasive breast cancer is treated with various modalities which include:
- Surgery
- Chemotherapy
- Radiotherapy
- Hormonal treatment
- Targeted therapy.

The sequence and possible usefulness of each of these modalities will depend upon the clinical stage of the disease and results of IHC of the tumor tissue.

Surgical Treatment

The aim of breast cancer surgery should be:
- Complete resection of the primary tumor with negative margins
- Decrease the risk of local recurrences as much as possible
- Acquire prognostic information through pathologic staging of the tumor and axillary lymph nodes.

Surgical treatment comprises of treatment of breast containing tumor and management of ipsilateral axillary lymph nodes. Breast surgeries commonly employed are either wide local excision of the breast lump breast conserving surgery (BCS) or mastectomy [modified radical mastectomy (MRM)].

Absolute contraindication to BCS are:
- Patient is pregnant as that will preclude the use of adjuvant radiotherapy
- Multicentric tumors
- Diffuse suspicious microcalcifications
- Persistently positive margins
- A history of previous therapeutic irradiation to the breast region.

Margin Status Recommendations Post BCS for DCIS and Invasive Ductal Carcinoma

- To ensure complete excision of the DCIS associated with diffuse microcalcification, detected by mammography, the excised specimen should be analyzed by specimen radiography.
- The NCCN (2018) recommends a positive margin for DCIS or invasive stage I, II, and selected cases of stage III breast cancer, treated by BCS, as one with "ink on tumor". To ensure no ink on tumor, either re-excision if feasible should be done till no tumor with ink is achieved, or proceed to mastectomy. Quantitative description of close margin for pure DCIS treated with BCS and adjuvant EBRT is 2 mm or less and is associated

with increased incidence of ipsilateral breast tumor recurrence. However, margins wider than 2 mm do not improve outcome.

Modified Radical Mastectomy

The first mastectomy based on scientific principles was radical mastectomy done by Halsted in 1889. It entailed the resection of the affected breast along with underlying pectoralis major muscle, axillary lymph nodes, supraclavicular lymph nodes, and ipsilateral internal mammary lymph nodal chain.

The switch to MRM occurred when it was recognised that treatment failure after breast surgery is usually because of systemic dissemination of cancer cells before surgery and not an inadequate operative procedure. It was first popularised by Patey in 1948. MRM was a big leap over Radical Mastectomy as pectoralis major muscle was not resected unless it was infiltrated. Neck nodes and internal mammary lymph nodes were also left untouched.

Axillary Lymph Nodal Staging

Regional nodal dissection is performed for:
- Staging
- Prognosis
- Regional control
- Improving survival.

Axillary lymph nodal staging is done either upfront axillary lymph node dissection (ALND) or after SLNB. Patients presenting with axillary nodal enlargement should be subjected to image-guided FNA or core needle biopsy. Patients with positive lymph nodes will need ALND. Patients with clinically free axilla should be considered for SLNB. For sentinel lymph node (SLN) mapping, injections can be administered peritumoral, subareolar or subdermal. For SLN mapping, dyes used can be isosulfan blue or methylene blue. However, radiolabeled sulfur colloid is also used frequently.

Identified SLN is subjected to multilevel H&E staining. Cytokeratin IHC is reserved for equivocal cases only. Patients with positive SLN should be considered for ALND. Axillary level III should be considered only in case of gross disease at level I and II.

According to the American Society of Clinical Oncology (ASCO) guidelines, sentinel lymph node biopsy should not be performed in patients with any of the following:
- Locally advanced invasive breast cancer
- Inflammatory breast cancer
- DCIS (when breast-conserving surgery is planned)
- Pregnant patient.

The ASCO recommendations regarding ALND in patients who have undergone sentinel lymph node biopsy are as follows:
- Axillary lymph node dissection should not be performed in women with no SLN metastases.
- In most cases, ALND should not be performed in women with one to two metastatic SLNs who are planning to undergo breast-conserving surgery with whole-breast radiotherapy.
- Axillary lymph node dissection should be offered to women with SLN metastases who will be undergoing mastectomy.

Adjuvant Therapy in Early Breast Invasive Cancer

Adjuvant treatment of breast cancer is designed to treat micrometastatic disease. Adjuvant treatment for breast cancer involves radiation therapy and systemic therapy (including a variety of chemotherapeutic, hormonal, and biologic agents). Chemotherapy takes the precedence over radiotherapy in all cases where both are to be incorporated in adjuvant settings. In early-stage breast cancer, tumor gene-expression assays can be used to determine the likelihood of recurrence and thus the potential benefit of adjuvant chemotherapy.

Postlumpectomy Radiation Therapy

Adjuvant radiation therapy after BCS eradicates local subclinical residual disease and reduces local recurrence rates by approximately 75%.

Radiotherapy can be delivered by either conventional EBRT or by partial breast irradiation (PBI). EBRT delivers a dose of 50–55 Gy over 5–6 weeks to breast followed by booster dose of 10–16 Gy to the tumor site in the breast. START trial confirmed that 3-week hypofractionated adjuvant radiotherapy (40 Gy in 15 fractions over 3 weeks) is as effective and safe as the international standard 5-week regimen (50 Gy in 25 fractions) for women with early-stage breast cancer following primary surgery.

Partial breast irradiation delivers large fraction radiation dose sizes twice daily for 5 days with a low risk of radiation associated late effects in early-stage breast cancer after breast-conserving surgery.

The American Society of Breast Surgeons (ASBrS) recommends the following selection criteria when patients are being considered for treatment with accelerated PBI.
- Age more than or equal to 45 years for invasive cancer and more than or equal to 50 years for DCIS
- Invasive ductal carcinoma or DCIS
- Total tumor size (invasive and DCIS) less than or equal to 3 cm
- Negative microscopic surgical margins of excision
- Sentinel lymph node negative.

According to two major studies (TARGIT-A trial and ELIOT study), single-dose radiotherapy delivered during or soon after surgery for breast cancer is a viable alternative to conventional EBRT in selected patients who are at low risk for local recurrence.

Postmastectomy Radiation Therapy

According to ASCO, the criteria recommended for postmastectomy radiation therapy are:
- Positive postmastectomy margins
- Primary tumors more than 5 cm
- Positive axillary lymph nodes.

The NCCN guidelines strongly recommends radiation to ipsilateral chest wall, infrascapular and supraclavicular regions, ipsilateral axillary bed, and ipsilateral internal mammary nodes in patients with more than 4 positive lymph nodes. For patients with 1–3 positive axillary lymph nodes irradiation to ipsilateral chest wall and axillary bed is recommended. In patients with negative nodes, tumor less than 5 cm and clear margin 1 mm or more, no post mastectomy irradiation is needed. However patients with negative axillary nodes but with tumors of 5 cm or more in size and/or margins positive or less than 1 mm of clear margin, ipsilateral chest wall irradiation is advocated. In the AMAROS trial, which involved patients with cT1-2N0 breast cancer up to 5 cm, and clinically node-negative axillae. They underwent either breast conservation or mastectomy with SLN mapping. According to the results of this trial axillary radiotherapy was found to be a better treatment option than ALND in women with a positive SLN.

Adjuvant Systemic Therapy

It is based on risk of relapse of disease and sensitivity to the treatment, i.e. ER, PR, and HER2. It is also based on the toxicity of the treatment and comorbidity. Many gene-based assays such as 21 gene assay and 70 gene signatures can predict prognosis in terms of local and distant recurrence and survival.

Axillary lymph node negative tumors:
- Breast tumors of less than 0.5 cm have favorable outcome and do not benefit from chemotherapy. However endocrine therapy may be used in ER-positive patients to reduce the chances of contralateral breast tumors.
- Patients with invasive ductal and lobular carcinomas of more than 0.5 cm are categorized into low-risk and the high-risk ones having unfavorable prognostic features which include angiolymphatic invasion, high nuclear grade, high histologic grade, and HER2 positive and negative hormonal receptor status. Need for adjuvant therapy in low-risk group will need balancing between the expected absolute risk reduction and therapy induced toxicity.

- For breast tumors greater than 1 cm chemotherapy is strongly recommended.

Axillary lymph node positive tumors: They are usually the candidates for chemotherapy. Patients with hormone receptor (HR) positive tumors should be considered for endocrine therapy irrespective of patient age, lymph node status, and whether chemotherapy is administered or not.

Tamoxifen is used in both pre- and postmenopausal breast malignancies. NCCN panel recommends in postmenopausal women tamoxifen for 2–3 years followed by aromatase inhibitor to complete 5 cycles of adjuvant endocrine therapy. Other option is tamoxifen for 5–6 years followed by aromatase inhibitor for 5 years. Tamoxifen alone for 10 years is also strongly recommended.

For premenopausal women, NCCN panel recommends:
- Five year tamoxifen with or without ovarian suppression
- Five year aromatase inhibitor with ovarian suppression.

Adjuvant Cytotoxic Chemotherapy

The preferred regimens include:
- Dose dense doxorubicin and cyclophosphamide (AC) with dose dense sequential paclitaxel
- Dose dense doxorubicin and cyclophosphamide followed by sequential weekly paclitaxel
- Docetaxel plus cyclophosphamide (TC).

Other regimens include:
- Doxorubicin and cyclophosphamide (AC)
- Epirubicin and cyclophosphamide (EC)
- Cyclophosphamide methotrexate fluorouracil (CMF)
- Doxorubicin and cyclophosphamide with sequential docetaxel every 3 weeks
- Doxorubicin and cyclophosphamide with sequential weekly paclitaxel
- 5-fluorouracil, epirubicin, and cyclophosphamide/cyclophosphamide, epirubicin, and 5-fluorouracil (FEC/CEF) followed by docetaxel or weekly paclitaxel.

Based on the NSABP B 36 results, NCCN panel excluded FEC/CEF and FAC/CAF [5-fluorouracil, doxorubicin, and cyclophosphamide/cyclophosphamide, doxorubicin (adriamycin), and 5-fluorouracil] regimens as an option of adjuvant therapy as women on these regimens experienced worse quality-of-life at 6 months of life and high chances of chemotherapy-induced amenorrhea.

Adjuvant HER2-Targeted Therapy

It is recommended in HER2 positive tumors. Trastuzumab is a humanized monoclonal antibody. Doxorubicin and cyclophosphamide followed by paclitaxel with trastuzumab for 1 year commencing with the first dose of paclitaxel is the preferred HER2 targeting adjuvant regimens. Various trials have shown incorporation of HER2-targeted therapy in patients with HER2-positive breast tumors significantly improved DFS and OS.

LOCALLY ADVANCED BREAST CANCERS

It is a clinical subset of patients where the invasive breast cancer on clinical and imaging evaluation is advanced but confined to the breast and ipsilateral axillary lymph nodes only. Locally advanced breast cancer (LABC) is staged as stage III. It is again also substaged as:
- Operable LABC where upfront surgery can achieve negative margins.
- Inoperable LABC where initial surgical resection cannot obtain negative resection margins. They will require presurgical systemic therapy to downstage the tumor.

INFLAMMATORY BREAST CANCER

Inflammatory breast cancer is a clinical diagnosis. It presents with signs and symptoms akin to an inflammation. However the mass is not usually well appreciated and even if it is appreciated the true extent of the disease is usually greater than is apparent on physical examination. Incidence of IBC is 1–2% of all breast cancers. IBC tends to occur at a younger age than LABC. Pathologically, IBC are usually HR negative and HER2 positive.

PRINCIPLES OF PREOPERATIVE SYSTEMIC THERAPY

Candidates for preoperative systemic therapy are:
- Inoperable breast cancers:
  - Inflammatory breast cancer
  - Matted N2 axillary nodes
  - N3 nodes
  - T4 tumors.
- Operable disease:
  - Large primary tumor relative to breast size
  - With node positive disease likely to become negative with pre-operative therapy.

Patients where extent of disease cannot be delineated, e.g. with extensive in situ disease, poorly delineated tumors, preoperative systemic therapy is not advisable.

Preoperative therapy can:
- Downstage the tumor and render an inoperable tumor into an operable one.

- It will increase the feasibility of breast conservation therapy.
- It also offers us an opportunity to assess the response of tumor to the therapeutic agent.

Pathological complete response to preoperative treatment is associated extremely favorable DFS and OS and this association is particularly found in triple negative breast cancers. In general chemotherapeutic regimens recommended in preoperative setting are the same as in adjuvant settings. Patients with ER positive disease and comorbidities and low risk luminal disease may be considered for preoperative endocrine therapy. Patients with HER2-positive disease should receive regimens incorporating trastuzumab for at least 9 weeks before surgery. Patients with disease equal to or greater than T2 or having nodal disease equal to or greater than N1 may receive regimens incorporating pertuzumab. When using preoperative chemotherapy all treatment should preferably be administered before surgery. Tumor response should be assessed regularly by clinical examination and imaging. Any indication of progressive disease should warrant change in chemotherapy regimen or proceed to surgery.

BREAST RECONSTRUCTION FOLLOWING SURGERY

All patients undergoing surgery for breast malignancy should be made aware of breast reconstruction options. However, the need for breast reconstruction should not override the fact that delivery of appropriate and timely surgical treatment is more important and also breast reconstruction should not interfere in the efficacy of further future treatment. Breast reconstruction may utilize breast implants or autologous tissue transfers or both. Reconstruction can be immediate, delayed or staged. Immediate reconstruction is not however recommended in case of mastectomy for IBCs in view of the aggressive nature of the disease and high chances of recurrences.

Follow-up Post-treatment in Stage I to III

It includes:
- History and physical examinations every 4–6 months for 5 years and then annually.
- Annual mammogram.
- The NCCN guidelines suggest that in absence of clinical signs and symptoms suggestive of recurrent or metastatic disease, laboratory and imaging investigations are unnecessary with no advantage of survival or improved chances of palliation. MRI of breast is however indicated in patients who carry greater than 20% lifetime risk of developing breast cancer.
- Yearly gynecological assessment of patients taking tamoxifen.
- Symptomatic management includes treatment of hot flushes by venlafaxine and management of concurrent depression.

- Educating patient regarding arm lymphedema, its monitoring, and management.
- Assuring the assessment of adherence of patient to ongoing medication regimens, including endocrine therapy.
- Young women, post-treatment may regain their premenopausal status. They should use birth control methods other than hormonal ones.
- Patients using aromatase inhibitors should have periodical bone mineral density determination. Premenopausal patients with severe osteoporosis should receive 6 monthly infusion of bisphosphonates, e.g. zoledronic acid. Denosumab has been found to reduce significantly the risk of pathological fractures in postmenopausal ladies.

Prophylactic Mastectomy

It can be considered in women who are at a very high risk of having breast cancer and most often it is because of the certain genetic mutations that puts a woman at very high risk. It includes:
- Strong family history of breast and/or ovarian cancer
- Pathogenic mutation in *BRCA1* or *BRCA2*
- High-penetrance mutation in another gene associated with breast cancer risk (e.g. *TP53*, *PTEN*).

Bilateral risk-reduction mastectomy decreases the risk of developing breast cancer by at least 90% in women at moderate to high risk and in those with known *BRCA1/2* mutations.

METASTATIC/RECURRENT BREAST CANCER

Patients presenting with metastasis or recurrent disease need re-evaluation by:
- History of disease, signs, and symptoms
- CBC and LFT
- Contrast-enhanced CT of chest and abdomen
- Bone scan
- Biopsy documentation of the metastasis at presentation or first recurrence, if possible.

The NCCN panel consensus is that FDG (fluorodeoxyglucose) PET/CT is optional and is most useful where standard imaging results are suspicious or equivocal. Biopsy of the metastasis or recurrent disease ensures its diagnosis, tumor histology, and allow for biomarker assessment (ER, PR, and HER2). Discordance of the receptor status of the primary and recurrent breast tumors is known.

Management of Local Recurrence

Local recurrence in patients having undergone mastectomy followed by radiotherapy previously, should be treated by surgical excision, provided it does not entail extremely radical resections. The aim of resection should be to obtain clear resection margins. Unresectable recurrences should be treated with radiotherapy if it was not used previously.

Patients with local recurrences, post initial BCS should undergo total mastectomy and the level I and II axillary dissection if was not done previously.

After treating local recurrences patients should receive limited duration systemic therapy—chemotherapy and/or endocrine therapy. Systemic therapy improves survival and quality-of-life but is not curative.

Patients of carcinoma breast with local recurrence or metastases can be stratified for treatment on the basis of presence or absence of skeletal metastases. Bisphosphonates (zoledronic acid and pamidronate) and denosumab (inhibits RANK Ligand, an activator of osteoclast function) are very effective in preventing skeletal-related events, e.g. bone pains, bone fractures, spinal cord compression, and hypercalcemia. Both bisphosphonates and denosumab can cause osteonecrosis of jaw, especially in patients with underlying poor orodental health or dental procedure during treatment.

Endocrine Therapy in Metastatic or Recurrent Disease

Premenopausal patients without the exposure to previous antiestrogens should receive selective ER modulators alone. However, those exposed to the endocrine therapy within the last 1 year receive the second-line therapy in the form of ovarian ablation or suppression followed by endocrine therapy.

Various endocrine therapies for metastatic or recurrent postmenopausal women include:
- Nonsteroidal aromatase inhibitors (anastrozole and letrozole)
- Steroidal aromatase inhibitors (exemestane)
- Serum ER modulators (tamoxifen and toremifene)
- Estrogen receptor down regulators (fulvestrant)
- Progestins (megestrol acetate).

New combination therapies have now come in use, e.g.:
- Palbociclib with fulvestrant or letrozole
- Exemestane with everolimus.
  Palbociclib is a highly selective inhibitor of CDK4/6 kinase activity.

According to the NCCN guidelines combination of palbociclib with letrozole is the first line of chemotherapy option in postmenopausal women with HR-positive and HER2-negative metastatic breast cancer. Palbociclib with fulvestrant is also the first option in HR-positive HER2-negative metastatic breast cancer in postmenopausal or premenopausal women receiving ovarian suppression with luteinizing hormone-releasing hormone (LHRH) agonist.

Cytotoxic Chemotherapy for Metastatic or Recurrent Breast Cancer

Its indications are:
- Hormone receptor-negative patients with disease not localized to bone or soft tissue only and associated with symptomatic visceral metastasis
- Hormone receptor-positive patients resistant to endocrine therapy.

Combination chemotherapy is preferable to single cytotoxic agents for favorable responses. Chemotherapeutic agents used in metastatic settings are the same as those used in adjuvant settings of stage I to III invasive breast carcinomas. Since sequential responses are experienced with the cytotoxic agents, they should be used sequentially either as single agents or in combination therapy. Failure to elicit response after three sequential chemotherapy regimens or Eastern Cooperative Oncology Group (ECOG) level of 3 or greater is an indication for supportive care only.

HER2-Targeted Therapy in Metastatic or Recurrent Breast Cancer

It is recommended in patients with HER2-positive tumors. The NCCN panel recommends combination of trastuzumab and pertuzumab with docetaxel as the most preferred regimen in patients with HER2-positive metastatic or recurrent breast malignancy.

FERTILITY AND BIRTH CONTROL

All premenopausal ladies who desire to be pregnant should be referred to the fertility specialists before the start of systemic therapy (chemotherapy or hormonal treatment). They may need oocyte or embryo preservation. Many females start menses within 2 years after completion of therapy. However, menses and fertility are not inter-related as either of them can be present in absence of other and vice-versa. Pregnancy should be avoided while undergoing radiotherapy or systemic therapy. Trials have shown that ovarian function can be preserved in premenopausal ladies with ER-negative breast cancers by the administration of gonadotropin-releasing hormone agonists. There is no contraindication to breast feeding post BCS.

CONCLUSION

- Breast cancers are a leading cause of cancer related deaths in females. Any symptom related to breasts should be taken seriously and all asymptomatic women should subject themselves for screening at the recommended ages.
- Initial assessment of breast cancer is by triple assessment which includes Clinical examination, imaging and pathological evaluation. Further

evaluation includes the investigations for assessing clinical staging. Immunohistochemistry (IHC) and molecular profiling assays can predict the need for further modes of treatment after surgery.
- Preinvasive breast tumors are treated by surgery, radiotherapy and hormonal treatment. In early breast cancers chemotherapy and targeted therapy may also be needed. Locally advanced breast cancers usually require upfront systemic therapies followed by surgery and radiotherapy. Breast reconstruction awareness should be made available to all patients undergoing surgery.

SUGGESTED READING

1. ASCO Clinical Practice Guidelines updates.
2. DeVita, Hellman, and Rosenberg's Cancer: Principles & Practice of Oncology.
3. NCC guidelines for Breast Cancer.

Index

Page numbers followed by *b* refer to box; *f* refer to figure; *fc* refer to flow chart; and *t* refer to table respectively.

A

Abdominal
   adhesion 59
   examination 55, 69, 125
Abortions
   clinical care of 161
   complications of 163
      hemorrhage 163
      incomplete abortion 163
      infections 163
      ongoing pregnancy 163
   medical methods of 162, 162*b*
   unsafe 156
Acanthosis nigricans 113
Actinomyces israelii 25
Actinomycete 100
Adenocarcinoma 212
   cervix 210
Adenomyosis 44, 48
   in uterus 50
   uteri 51*f*
Adenosquamous carcinoma 213
Adhesions 59
   removal of 136
Adipose cells 110
Adipose tissue
   expandability theory 110
   hypotrophy of 110
Adnexal mass 60
Adominal examination 94
Adrenal
   androgens 2
   disorders 112
   hyperplasia, congenital 11
Adrenarche 4
   stages of 5*f*
Aerobic organisms 25
   gram-negative 25
   gram-positive 25
Alpha-fetoprotein 93
Alzheimer's disease, prevention of 196

Amenorrhea 134
American College of Obstetricians and Gynecologists Practice guidelines 98*t*
American College of Radiology Imaging Network 170
American Heart Association Guidelines 197
American Joint Committee on Cancer Stages 168
American Society for Reproductive Medicine 107, 198
American Society of Breast Surgeons 241
American Society of Clinical Oncology 240
Amitriptyline 64
Amphetamine analog 115
Ampicillin-sulbactam, combination of 103
Anaerobic organisms 25
   gram-negative 26
   gram-positive bacilli 25
   gram-positive cocci 25
Anastrozole 247
Androgen Excess Society 107, 108
Androgen secreting tumors 11
Androstenedione, production of 2
Anorexia nervosa 6
Antara Program 146
Antifibrinolytics 40
Antimineralocorticoid action 141
Anti-Müllerian hormone 18
Antioxidants 137
Antiprogesterone drug 86
Antral follicle count 128, 129
Apolipoprotein A1 96
Apolipoprotein B levels 16
Asherman's syndrome 46
Assisted Reproductive Technology 128, 136, 138
Atrophic vaginitis 26

Atrophy 186, 191
Augmentation cystoplasty 75
Axillary lymph node 244
    staging 240
    dissection 240
    negative tumors 242
    positive tumors 243
Azithromycin 33, 104
Azoospermia 131, 133, 137, 138

B

Back pain, isolated 61*f*
Bacterial morphology, types of 30
Bacterial vaginosis 26, 28, 34, 99
    risk factors 28
    treatment regimen of 30*b*
Bacteroides 26, 30, 100
Bariatric surgery 115
Barrier contraception 149
Basal body temperature measurement 127
Behavioral therapy 65, 73
Benign breast tumors 145
Benign ovarian
    cysts 90, 145
    neoplasm 91
Benign pubertal variants 11
Beta-2 glycoprotein 96
Bicornuate uterus 51
Bifidobacterium 25
Biliopancreatic diversion 115
Biochemical markers 182
Biomarker, assessment of 246
Birth control 248
Bladder pain syndrome 67, 77, 79
    diagnosis 77
    treatment 77
Bladder syndrome 77
Bladder training 73
Bleeding
    after menopause 186
    causes of 186
        anticoagulant therapy 189
        atrophy 186
        cancer 188
        diseases in adjacent organs 189
        endometrial hyperplasia 187
        fibroid uterus 188
        herbal and dietary supplements 189
        infections 189
        polyps 187
        postmenopausal hormone therapy 188
        postradiation therapy 189
    loss, heavy 151
    per vaginam 151, 189
Blood
    borne metastasis 213
    hormone concentrations 4*t*
    pressure 143
    sugar fasting 125
Body mass index 11, 37
Bone mineral density 151, 199
Botox injections 75
Botulinum toxin 64
Botulinum toxoid 64
BRCA-related breast cancers 178
Breast anatomy 165, 166*f*
Breast cancer 167, 177, 197
    classification for 233
    clinical examination 230
    diagnosis of 179
    evaluation of 230
    frequency of 180
    further clinical staging 232
    genetic predisposition to 177
    HER2 testing 232
    histologic grade 236
    histological, types of 168
    histology 231
    locally advanced 233, 244
    management of 230
    metastatic 233, 246, 248
    molecular profiling assays 237
    recurrent 246, 248
    risk assessment tool 167
    risk factors 177
    screening 169, 178
        by imaging 178
        core needle biopsy 171
        examination by clinician 178
        fine-needle aspiration biopsy 171
        guidelines for women 171*t*
        magnetic resonance imaging 171

mammography 169
self and clinical assessment 169
self-breast examination 169
self-examination of 178
specimens 232
stage grouping 237
surgery 239
surveillance 165
symptoms 230
treatment 168
Breast changes 165, 166
Breast conservation surgery 238, 239
Breast imaging reporting and data system 170, 170*t*
Breast invasive cancer, adjuvant therapy in early 241
Breast malignancy
early stage 233
evaluation of 230
following surgery 245
Breast, pathologic lesions of 167
Breast, self-examination of 79*f*
Breast tenderness 86
Breast tissue 166
Breast tumor 231, 232
management of preinvasive 238
Bromocriptine 134
Bulking agents 74
Bullous edema 211

C

Cabergoline 134
Cancer antigen 125 182, 183, 225
breast 209
Cancer cervix
epidemiology of 209
types of 212
Cancer, family history of 38
Candida albicans 26
Candida with budding 30*f*
Candidal infection 33
Carcinogens mechanism of 209
Carcinoma 93
cervix uteri 211
cervix, features of 210
in breast parenchyma 234
invasive 211

ovary 205*t*
undifferentiated 204
Cardiovascular
disease 21, 22, 152
risk for 18
examination 69
system 199
Carnett's test 62*f*
Cefotaxime 104
Cefotetan 103
Cefoxitin 103
Ceftizoxime 104
Ceftriaxone 103
Celecoxib 56
Centchroman 146
Center for Disease Control and Prevention 105, 163
guidelines 104
Central Drug Standard Control Organization of India 86
Central nervous system 1, 17
lesion 10
Cerazette 144
Cervical
cancer 59, 175, 184, 209, 217, 217*t*
by stage, treatment of 218
during pregnancy 219
early-stage 216
recurrent 219
risk factors of 175
screening 176
frequency of 176
problems associated with sampling 176
caps 163
discharge 163
motion tenderness 100
polyps-cervical malignancy 26
screening 82
stenosis 51
stromal invasion 216
stump, cancer of 219
Chemoradiation 218
Chemotherapy
for advanced disease 218
use of 218
Chhaya 146
Chlamydia trachomatis 99, 100, 101, 209

Chlamydiasis 33
    recommendation for treatment of 33*b*
Chlormadinone acetate 143
Cholinergic agonist 77
Chronic immune suppression 209
Clear cell carcinoma 204
Climacteric 20
Clindamycin 103
    cream 30
Clomiphene citrate 118, 134
Clostridium 25
Clotrimazole cream 31, 33
Clue cells 29*f*
Coccobacillus 32
Coelomic epithelium 91
Cognitive behavioral therapy 226
Coital frequency 124
Colorectal carcinoma 145
Colposcopy 177*f*, 210
Combined oral contraceptive 141, 145, 153
    pills 42, 141, 142
    progestin, used in 143*t*
Comorbid depression 65
Condom 142
Congenital heart disease 195
Conjugated equine estrogens 199
Connective tissue atrophy 21, 22
Contraception
    how to start 143*t*
    in medical disorders 149
    making right choices 141
    methods of 148, 150*t*
Contraceptive
    choices and efficacy 141
    efficacy: 1*st* year of use 142*t*
    in women with medical disorders 153*t*
    methods 141
    pills 142
        constituents of 144*t*
    emergency 145
    use 152*f*
    vaginal ring 142, 148
Copper intrauterine device 148, 149
Copper T 142
Cord stromal tumors 90
Cornual block 136
Coronary intervention 196
Cough-Stress test 70
Craniopharyngiomas 6
Cushing's syndrome 22, 108
Cyclic norethisterone 43
Cyclophosphamide 243
Cyproterone acetate 143
Cyst, functional 91*f*
Cystic breast lumps 231
Cystic fibrosis transmembrane receptor 133
Cystoscopy 76
Cysts with clomiphene citrate 119
Cytochrome P450-17 109
Cytoreduction 222
Cytotoxic chemotherapy 248

D

Danazol 43
Decapeptyl 85
Deep endometriosis 59
Dehydroepiandrosterone 4, 114
    sulfate 16, 114
Deoxyribo-nucleic acid defects 132
Depomedroxyprogesterone acetate 142, 151, 153
Depression 153
Dermoid cyst, cut section image of 92, 92*f*
Desmopressin 44
Detrusor
    overactivity 75
    sphincter dyssynergia 76
Diet 114
Digital mammography 170
Dilatation and curettage 16
Diphenhydramine hydrochloride 78
Diphtheroids 25
Disease in
    bladder 189
    bowel 186, 189
    colon 186
    control and prevention 103
    urethra 186, 189
Disorders ovulation of 133
Distal block 136

DNA methyltransferase inhibitor 201
Docetaxel plus cyclophosphamide 243
Donor insemination 127
Dopamine
    agonists 121
    receptor agonist 134
Doxorubicin
    and cyclophosphamide 243
    plus cisplatin 224
Doxycycline 33, 103
Drospirenone 141
Drug administration 225
Dual-energy X-ray absorptiometry 19
Ductal carcinoma in situ 168, 233, 238
    treatment of 238
Duloxetine chloride 73
Duodenal switch 115
Dysfunctional uterine bleeding 37
Dysmenorrhea 49
    congestive 55
    etiology 50
        diagnosis 55
            primary dysmenorrhea 50
            secondary dysmenorrhea 50
        symptoms 54
        treatment 56
    incidence of 147
    membranous 57
    prevalence 49
    primary 56
    secondary 57
    treatment
        medical management 56
        surgical treatment 56
    types of 49
Dyspareunia 196
Dysuria 80

E

Eastern Cooperative Oncology Group 248
Ectocervix 175
Ectopic pregnancy 99, 145, 147
Electromyography 72
Embryonal cell, types of 93
Endocervical
    cancers 210

sample 62
smear 28
Endocrine disease 22
Endocrine therapy in
    metastatic disease 247
    recurrent disease 247
Endocrine umbrella 202
Endodermal
    ablation 45
    aspiration 38
    biopsy 19, 126
    carcinoma 17, 26, 59, 93, 113, 145, 183, 192, 221, 222
        diagnosis of 222
        epidemiology 221
        histologic types of 221
        histopathology 221
        hysteroscopy of 189f
        risk factors 222
        staging and treatment 222
            chemotherapy-related toxicities 225
            follow-up post-treatment 224
            pattern of recurrence 225
            prognosis 227
            surgical treatment 222
        survivors 226
        treatment for 227
    changes 19
    histopathology of 19
    hyperplasia 19, 113, 186, 189, 192
    laser interstitial thermal therapy 47
    neoplasm 222
    polyp in uterus 52f
    protection 198
    sampling 38
    sinus tumors 93
    thickness 19, 38, 196
Endometrioid tumors 92
Endometriomas 90
Endometriosis 50, 55, 77, 134, 181
Endometriotic lesion on peritoneum 50f
Endometrium 45, 199
    carcinoma staging and treatment of 227
Endometroid carcinoma 204
Endomyometrial surface 46
Enterobacter 25

Enterobius vermicularis infestation 26
Enterococcus faecalis 25
Enzyme-linked immunosorbent assay 28, 34
Epididymovasostomy 138
Epirubicin 243
Epithelial cell carcinoma 90
Epithelial ovarian cancer 204
    chemotherapy in 207
    prognostic variables for 206
Epithelial ovarian tumor, different types of 206*t*
Erythrocyte sedimentation rate 62
Erythromycin ethylsuccinate 33
Escherichia coli 25, 100
Estradiol 128
    level of 17, 201
    progesterone 12
    ratio of 137
    valerate 144
Estrogen 196, 198
    deficiency 186, 193
    deprivation 77
    metabolism 201
    replacement therapy 226
        newer developments 200
    use of 196
Estrogen-progesterone therapy 196
Estrogen-progestin, combination of 200
Ethamsylate 40
Ethinylestradiol 147
Etonogestrel implant 142
Eubacterium 25
Exercise 115
Exogenous androgen intake 108
External-beam radiotherapy 238
Extraurethral incontinence 68

F

Fallopian tube 136
    carcinoma in 26
Febrile morbidity 215
Federation of Gynecology and Obstetrics 222
Female
    external genitalia 184
    partner, evaluation of 124
    sterilization, standards for 152
Ferriman-Gallwey scoring 37

Fertile period, knowledge of 124
Fertility 248
    awareness-based method 142
    preservation 227
Fetal genes 110
Fibristal 86
Fibrocystic disease of breast 145
Fibroids 80-89
    classification 81
    close insight 80
    diagnosis 81
    hysteroscopy of 188*f*
    in uterus, different sites of 51*f*
    management of 82
        asymptomatic 82
        symptomatic 82
        types of 88*fc*
    risk factors 80
    signs and symptoms 80
    ultrasonography of 188
    uterus 186
Fibroprist 86
Filling cystometry 72
Finasteride 117
Fine-needle aspiration cytology 231
Fistula 68
    surgical treatment of 75
Fitz-Hugs-Curtis syndrome 100
Florid discharge 100
Fluorodeoxyglucose 246
Flutamide 117
Follicle-stimulating hormone 2, 4, 8, 16, 141
Food and Drug Administration 85*t*, 170, 196
    guidelines for conservative procedures 46
Foreign body 26
Forniceal tenderness 60, 100
Fragile X syndrome 15, 130
Fulvestrant 247
Fungal infection 30
    treatment of 31
    treatment regimen of 31*b*
Fusobacterium 26

G

Gabapentine 64
Gait assessment 69

Galactorrhea 10, 113
Gamma-aminobutyric acid 64
Gardnerella vaginalis 30
Gastrointestinal carcinomas 90
Genetic
    assessment 130
    counseling 133
    predisposition 109
    testing 133
Genital
    causes 186
    examination 130
    organs, changes in 4
Gentamycin 103
Germ cell tumors 90, 92, 95
Germline mutations 178
Gestrinone 43
Glandular
    cells, atypical 177
    component 165
    tissue 165
Glassy cell carcinoma 213
Gonadal
    sex steroids 2
    stroma 91
Gonadotropin-releasing hormone 2, 63, 66
    agonists 13, 43, 45, 85, 135, 248
    releasing neurons 110
Gonadotropins 12, 120, 134
Gonorrhea 62
Gram staining 28
Granulosa cell tumors 10, 94
Granulosa cells of growing follicles 129
Growth hormone 3
Gynecologic Oncology Group 218, 224
Gynecological cancer
    different types of 174
    screening of 174
Gynecological screening 18
Gynecology Oncology Center 96
Gynecology outpatient department 24

H

Haemophilus 100
Hepatitis B virus 104
HER2-targeted therapy metastatic breast cancer 248
Herbal and dietary supplements 186

Hereditary nonpolyposis
    colon cancer 38
    colorectal cancer 227
Herpes simplex virus 28
Hirsutism
    case of 37
    management of 116
Hormonal
    analysis 132
    pills, use of 97
Hormonal therapy 43
    women on 18
Hormone replacement therapy 38
    increased risk of 18
    menopause 193
Hormones 56
Hot flushes, development of 20
Human
    chorionic gonadotropin 137
    epidermal growth factor 232
        receptor 2 168
    epididymis 95
        protein 4 182
    immunodeficiency virus 101
        evaluation of 125
    menopausal gonadotropin 120, 135
    papillomavirus 104, 175
Hydrodistention 78
Hydrogen peroxide 26
Hydronephrosis 60
Hydrosalpinx 136
Hyperandrogenic chronic anovulation 107
Hyperestrogenic status 80
Hypergonadotropic hypogonadism 6
Hyperparathyroidism 22
Hyperplasia
    hysteroscopy of 188*f*
    ultrasonography of 188*f*
Hyperprolactinemia 134
Hypogonadotropic hypogonadism 6, 112, 135, 137
Hypomenorrhea 111
Hypothalamic amenorrhea, severe 6
Hypothalamic-pituitary axis matures 36
Hypothalamic-pituitary-adrenal 109
Hypothalamic-pituitary-ovarian 1, 2, 2*fc*, 109

Hypothyroidism 126
Hysterectomy 214
Hysterosalpingography 54f
Hysteroscopy-guided sampling 38
Hysteroscopic myomectomy 83

I

Ibuprofen 56
Immunohistochemical investigations 231
Imperforate hymen 51
In vitro fertilization 126
Incontinence quality of life 69
Infection with human papillomavirus 209
Infertile couple
   clinical history 124
   hormonal evaluations 129
   investigations 125
      for female partner 128
   management of 124-139
   physical examination 125, 130
   postcoital test 129
   surgical management 137
   treatment of
      ejaculatory disorders 138
      male factor infertility 136
      specific disorders 133
      tubal factor infertility 136
Infertile male partner, investigations for 132
Infertility management of 117
Infertility unexplained 139
Infiltrating lobular carcinoma 231
Inflammatory
   bowel disease 59
   breast cancer 231, 244
Infraumbilical pain 61f
Inhibin levels 12
Injectable progesterone 41
Inoperable breast cancers 244
Inositols function 121
Internal orifice 49
International Federation of Gynecology and Obstetrics 36, 81, 205, 210
International Federation of Gynecology and Obstetrics Classification of leiomyomas 81b, 81f

International Ovarian Tumor Analysis 96, 96t
International Pelvic Pain Society 60
Interstitial cystitis 59, 60, 77
Intracavitary lesions 128
Intrauterine adhesions 51
Intrauterine conditioning 110
Intrauterine contraception device 26, 55, 66, 146, 149
   use of 28
Intrauterine device 51, 142, 143, 151, 154
   hormone releasing 145
Intrauterine fetal programming 109
Intrauterine insemination 126
Intrauterine malnutrition 110
Intrauterine system 153
Invasive breast cancer: early stage, treatment of 239
Invasive cancer of cervix 213
   management of 213, 214t
Invasive ductal carcinoma 239
Irritable bowel syndrome 59
Isolated premature
   adrenarche 11
   menarche 11
   thelarche 11

K

Kallmann syndrome 6, 135
Karyotyping 133
King's health questionnaire 69
Klebsiella 25, 100
Krukenberg's tumor 94

L

Lactate dehydrogenase 95
Lactic acid 26
Lactobacilli 21, 25, 100
Lactobacillus 24, 30
Lactobacillus species 99
Lamotrigine 64
Langerhans cell 6
Laparoscopic
   hysterectomy 83
   in infertility workup 127
   myomectomy 83, 83f, 84f
   nerve ablation 56

ovarian drilling 120, 134
radical hysterectomy 216
uterosacral nerve ablation 65
Laurence-Moon-Bardet-Biedl syndrome 6
Leiomyomas 44, 80
Leptin 3
Lesion size 216
Lesions in breast, types of 167
nonproliferative lesions 167
proliferative changes 167
proliferative lesions with atypia 167
Letrozole 118, 119, 247
Leukocyte protease inhibitor 26
Leukocytospermia 132
Leuprolide 43
Levofloxacin 33, 103
Levonorgestrel 66, 86, 144, 153, 200
intrauterine contraceptive device 63, 143
Levonorgestrel-releasing intrauterine device 145
Leydig cell tumors 10
Light amplification by stimulated emission of radiation 39
Liquid-based cytology 18, 28, 176*f*
Lobular carcinoma in situ 166, 233, 238
history of 168
Lorcaserin 115
Low-density lipoprotein 16
Lower segment cesarean section 54, 154
Lumpectomy 168
Lupride 85
Luteinizing hormone 2, 4, 16, 111
pattern of 1
releasing hormone 247
Lymph nodes 217, 223
Lymphadenectomy 215
Lymphatic metastasis 213
Lymphedema 226
Lymph-vascular space invasion 216
Lynch syndrome 181, 184, 227

M

Magnetic resonance imaging 62, 231
guided high-intensity focused ultrasound 48
Male and female barrier methods 148
Male partner
clinical history 130
evaluation of 130
investigations 131
Malignancy 46, 59, 186
high risk of 96
Malignant cells 235
Malignant germ cell neoplasm, management of 208
Malignant germ cell tumor 93*f*
Malignant ovarian
masses 96
neoplasm 93
primary 90
secondary 90
Malignant tumors 182
Malodorous vaginal discharge 28
Mammaprint assay 238
Mammogram, diagnostic 231
Mastectomy 168
Maternal morbidity 156
Mayer-Rokitansky-Küster-Hauser syndrome 6
McCune-Albright syndrome 11
Medical abortion 156
general practitioner 156
use of antibiotic for 161
Medical termination of pregnancy 156
Act, 1971 157, 160
Medroxyprogesterone 63, 196
acetate 41, 146
Medullary carcinoma 231
Mefenamic acid 40, 56
Megestrol acetate 247
Menopausal hormone therapy 197, 198
crisis of 194
fifth crisis 195
first crisis 194
fourth crisis 195
second crisis 194
third crisis 194
low-dose 199
rationality of low-dose 198
Menopausal symptoms 199, 201, 226
Menopause 15
and symptomatology 20
consequences of 21
diagnosis of 15
evaluation of women 18
markers 19
myth of 193

physiology 15
physiology 15
prediction of 18
status 183
symptomatology 15
Menorrhagia 45
Menstrual
   bleeding, heavy 43
   cycle 111, 166
   cycle 128
   disorders management of 116
   period 161
Mentally ill person 159
Metastases 234-236
Metformin 121
Methylation 201
Metronidazole 30
Metrorrhagia 111
Micronized purified flavonoid fractions 40
Microsatellite instability testing 227
Microsurgical epididymal sperm aspiration 138
Microwave endometrial ablation 39
Midluteal serum progesterone measurement 126
Midsegment block 136
Mifepristone 45, 86, 162
Migraine headaches with aura 153
Million women study 195
Mirabegron 74
Mirena® IUD 142, 146*f*
Mixed germ cell tumors 93
Mixed incontinence 68
Mobiluncus 30
Molecular testing 28
Monophasic pill 143
Mood disorders 21
Morbidity
   acute 218
   chronic 218
Morphology index 182
Mucinous
   carcinoma 231
   cystadenocarcinoma 204
   cystadenomas 90
Müllerian
   anomalies 128
   dysgenesis 6

Multilocular cysts 183
Musculoskeletal conditions 59
Mutation in
   MLH1 181
   BRCA2 180
Mycoplasma genitalium 100
Myocardial infarction 196
Myo-inositol 121
Myoma 89
   closure of 84*f*
   enucleation of 84*f*
   incision on 83*f*
Myomectomy 45, 48, 83

N

Naproxen 56
National Cancer Institute 167
National Center for Health Statistics 163
National Institute of Health 107, 108
Needle biopsy 231
Neisseria gonorrhoeae 32, 50, 99
   infection 26
   recommendation for 33*b*
Neodymiumyttrium aluminum garnet 47
Neoplasm of hypothalamic 6
Nerve entrapment in wall 59
Nerve-sparing radical hysterectomy 216
Nestorone 143
Neuroendocrine carcinoma 213
Neurogenic detrusor over activity 68
Neurological
   diseases 76
   examination 76
Neuromodulation 65, 75
Neuropathic pain 64
Neurophysiologic tests 72
Nexplanon radiopaque 147
Nocturia 74
Nocturnal enuresis 74
Nodal disease 245
Nomegestrol 143
Noncontraceptive reproductive benefits 145*t*
Nonepithelial ovarian cancer 207
Nongenital causes 186
Nonhysteroscopy procedures 47

Nonsteroidal
    anti-inflammatory drug 63, 45, 47, 56, 66, 87
    aromatase inhibitors 247
Noradrenaline 64
Norethisterone 41
Nortriptyline 64
Nucleic acid amplification test 101

O

Obese males with low testosterone 137
Obstetrics and gynecology, progress of 195
Ofloxacin 33
Oligoasthenoteratozoospermia, case of severe 127
Oligomenorrhea 111, 134
    common cause of 126
Oligozoospermia, severe 131
Omentum 223
Onco type Dx assay 237
Operable disease 244
Opioidergic 64
Opioids 64
Oral contraceptive 66
Oral contraceptive pill 116, 145
Oral glucose tolerance test 114
Oral progesterones 41
Orlistat 115
Osteoclast function, activator of 247
Osteoporosis 21, 198, 199
    effects of ultra-low transdermal estradiol 199
    low-dose estrogen patch for 199
    risk factors for the development of 22
Osteoprotection 197
Ovarian
    cancer 145, 180, 198, 204
        classification 204
        epithelial ovarian tumor 205
        global incidence of 198
        high-risk factors 205, 206
        histological, types of 204t
        incidence of 204
        management of 207
        risk factors 180
        statistics and screening of 181
        surgical procedures for ovarian 207
    cysts 10, 59, 61f, 147
        approach to patient 94
        case of 90-98
        conservative management for 97
        functional 90
    cystectomy 154
    diagnosis of 135
    dysmetabolic syndrome 107
    endometrioma 50
    failure
    fibroma 92
    function 20
    hyperstimulation syndrome 120
    malignancy 93
    markers 95
    mass, types of 90t
    neoplasm histological classification of 91t
    sequelae of 20
    tumors 10
Ovaries 4
Ovulation, confirm 126
Ovulatory
    disturbance 108
    function 134
    problem 126
Oxybutynin 74

P

Pad tests 70
Paget's disease 233
Palbociclib 247
Pap smear 18, 176f
Para-aortic lymph node
    evaluation 215
    metastasis 211, 215t
Paracervical block 47
Parametrial spread 217
Paraovarian cysts 90
Pelvic abscess 104
Pelvic congestion 59
Pelvic examination 69, 76, 125, 181
    bimanual 100
Pelvic inflammatory disease 46, 99, 105, 145, 147
    acute 50, 99
    clinical diagnosis 100

    endometrial biopsy 102
    follow-up 104
    imaging 101
    inpatient therapy 103
    inpatient treatment versus
       outpatient treatment 104
    laboratory diagnosis 101
    laparoscopy 102
    pathogenesis and microbiology 99
    surgical intervention 104
    treatment of 102
  chronic 50, 59
    long-term sequelae of 105
    risk factors for 99
Pelvic lymph node metastasis 211
Pelvic lymphadenectomy 215
Pelvic pain 63, 163
Pelvic pain
  chronic 58-66, 99, 105
    algorithm to manage 66*fc*
    causes of 59, 59*t*
    diagnostic test 62
    management of 63-64
    physical examination 60, 60*t*
    recurrence of 63
    syndrome, chronic 63*f*
Peptostreptococcus 25, 100
Per speculum examination 210
Perifimbrial adhesions 136
Perimenopause 36
Peripheral vascular disease 152
Peritubal adhesions 136
Pertuzumab 245
Pervaginal examination 55
pH of vaginal discharge 28
Phentermine extended release
    topiramate 115
Phentermine-topiramate 115
Pill chhaya 147
Pinworm 26
Pituitary
  adenomas 6
  gonadotropin 10
Polycystic ovarian
  disease 107, 181
  morphology 108
  syndrome 38, 80, 107-121, 126, 133

  age-wise manifestation of 112*f*
  clinical features 111
  criteria for defining 108*b*
  criteria in adolescence 108
  diagnosis in adolescence 109*b*
  different criteria 108
  enigma of 107
  etiology 109
  etiopathogenesis of 111*fc*
  examination in 113*b*, 114*b*
  management, lifestyle
      modification 114
  pathogenesis 110
  prevalence 109
  role of medicines 121
  ultrasound in 114*b*
Polymenorrhea 111
Polymerase chain reaction 34
Polyp 48, 51, 186, 191
Polyurethane female condoms 149
Positron emission tomography scan 231
Postabortion care 163
Postcoital bleed 60
Postejaculation urine analysis 133
Postlumpectomy radiation therapy 241, 242
Postmenopausal
  age group 26
  bleeding, management of 189
    examination 190
    investigations 190
    treatment 191
  hormone therapy 186, 191
  woman 97
Postpartum hemorrhage, severe 135
Postpartum intrauterine contraceptive
    devices 148
Postradiation therapy 186
Postvoid residual volume 70
Potassium hydroxide 34
  smear 28
Pouch of Douglas 100, 101
Preabortion care 161
Precocious puberty 9
  causes of 10
  diagnosis of 11
  laboratory diagnose 11

physical examination 11
    treatment 12
Pregabalin 64
Pregnancy 24, 46
    of gestational age 162
    on dopamine receptor 134
    with fibroids 81
Pregnant women 157
Preimplantation genetic diagnosis 133
Premarin 43
Premature ovarian failure 15, 135
    diagnosis of 23
Premenopausal women 243
Premenstrual
    phase of cycle 25
    syndrome 147
Prenatal androgen exposure 110
Prepubertal girls 26
Presacral neurectomy 56
Progesterones 41
Progestin 196, 198
Progestin-only pill 142, 143, 144, 152-154
Progestogen-only implant 147
Program for Approved Technology in
        Health 149
Progynova 200
Prolactin 129
Prophylactic mastectomy 246
Prostaglandin synthetase inhibitors 40
Proteus 25, 100
Pseudomonas species 25
Pubertal staging 11
Puberty 6, 25
Puberty
    abnormal 1
    changes of 3*fc*
    endocrinology in 2
    factors determining onset of 1
    mechanism 1
    normal 1
    precocious 10
Pubovaginal sling 74
Pudendal nerve
    stimulation 65
    terminal motor latency 72
Pulmonary
    disease, chronic 69
    embolus 215
    tuberculosis 100
Pyospermia 132

Q

Qlaira, advantages of 144
Quality of life measures 69
Quantity of intraductal component 232

R

Radiation
    cystitis 59
    exposure 166
    related gastrointestinal toxicity 226
    therapy 213
        primary 217
Radical
    hysterectomy 214
        complications of 215
    mastectomy, modified 239, 240
    surgery 192
    trachelectomy 214
Radiofrequency ablation 39
Radiographic density 165
Regional lymph node 234, 235
Registered Medical Practitioner 157
Reproductive age 36
Retrograde ejaculation 138
Retropubic urethropexy 74
Rh immunization 161
Rh typing 125
Rheumatoid arthritis 153
Risk malignancy index 96*t*
Rotterdam's European Society of Human
        Reproduction and Embryology
        107
Roux-en-Y gastric bypass 115
Royal College of Obstetricians and
        Gynecologists 58
    guidelines 97
Rudimentary horns 53

S

Sacral nerve blocks 65
Sacral nerve 65
Saline hysterosonography 128
Saline infusion sonohysterography 38
Salpingo-oophorectomy, bilateral 94
Sarcoma 213
    of uterus 188

Sclerosis, multiple 76
Sclerotic polycystic ovary syndrome 107
Scrotal ultrasound 132
Secrete human chorionic gonadotropin 93
Selective estrogen receptor modulators 43, 167
Selective progesterone receptor modulators 45, 88, 85
Semen
    analysis 131
    sample 131
Seminal fructose 132
Sentinel lymph node 240
    biopsy 238, 240
    evaluation 216
Septate uterus 51, 53
Serology of syphilis 101
Serotonin-norepinephrine reuptake inhibitors 64, 73
Serous cystadenocarcinoma 204
Serous cystadenomas 90
Sertoli cell 10
Sertoli-Leydig cell tumor 94
Sertraline 64
Serum
    androgen measurement 129
    anti-Müllerian hormone 128
    follicle stimulating hormone 128
    prolactin 134
    transaminases 86
Sex cord stromal tumor 92
Sex steroids, action of 110
Sex-hormone-binding globulin gene 109, 111
Sexual
    abuse 26
    arousal 24
    dysfunction 21, 124, 213, 226
    history 124
    partners, multiple 99, 209
    precocity 12
Sexually transmitted disease 26, 77, 99, 148
Sexually transmitted infection 100, 151
Sheehan's syndrome 135
Shigellosis 26
Sign of pelvic abscess 100
Single cell gel electrophoresis assay 133

Sleep 199
Society for Gynecologic Oncologists 224
Solid ovarian tumor 92
Solid tumors 92
Solifenacin succinate 74
Sonomammogram 231
Sperm
    chromatin structure assay 133
    concentration 131
    DNA fragmentation tests 133
    morphology 132
    motility 132
    vitality 132
Spermatogenesis either injection 137
Spermatozoa, absence of 131
Spinal cord stimulation 65
Spironolactone 117
Squamous cell cancer 212
Staphylococci 100
Staphylococcus aureus 25
Staphylococcus epidermidis 25
Stein-Leventhal syndrome 107
Sterilization permanent 152
Steroids 12
Stool examination 28
Streptococci 100
Streptococcus group 25
Stress incontinence 73
Stress incontinence surgical treatment for 74
Stress urinary incontinence 67
Stroke 153
Stromal cell tumors 92
Stromal cells proliferation 4
Submucosal fibroid 82*f*
Subserosal fibroid 82*f*
Supreme Court 158
Surgical sperm retrieval 138

T

Tamoxifen 118, 119, 134, 243
Tamoxifen therapy 38
Tanner staging 4*t*, 11
Tension free vaginal tape 74
Testicular failure 133
Testicular sperm
    aspiration 138
    extraction 138

Testosterone 12
Thalassemia screen 125
Thelarche 4
    stages of 5*f*
Thromboembolism 200
Thyroid
    disorders 134
    function tests 12
    gland 3
    profile 129
    stimulating hormone 8, 114
    swellings 113
Tibial nerve stimulation, posterior 65
Tinidazole 30
Tolteridine 74
Toremifene 247
Total cholesterol, higher levels of 16
Tranexamic acid 40, 87
Transcervical resection of endometrium 39, 45
Transcutaneous electrical nerve stimulation 56
Transdermal delivery systems 147
Transient incontinence 68
Transrectal ultrasound 132
Transthyretin 96
Transvaginal scan 19, 38, 181
Transvaginal ultrasonography 94, 126, 128
Transverse vaginal septum 53
Trichomonas vaginalis 32*f*
Trichomonial infection 34
Trichomoniasis 26, 31
    treatment regimen of 32*f*
Tricyclic antidepressants 64
Triiodothyronine 8
Tubal evaluation 127
    hysterosalpingo-contrast-sonography 127
    hysterosalpingography 127
Tubo-ovarian
    adhesions 102*f*
    complexes 90
    mass, ultrasound of 101*f*
    rupture of 100
Tumors
    endometrioid histology of 221
    markers 95, 181
    nonendometrioid histology of 221
Turner's syndrome 6, 15, 130

U

Ulipristal acetate 45, 85, 145
Ultrasound score 183
Uniconuate uterus 53, 53*f*
United States National Comprehensive Cancer Network 224
Ureterovaginal fistula 215
Urethral
    diverticula 77
    function 72
    mobility: Q-tip test 70
    sphincter contracts 76
Urge urinary incontinence 68
Urinary
    diversion 75
    frequency 80
    incontinence 67
        approach to patient with 69
        nonsurgical treatment 72
        risk factors for 69
        surgical treatment for 75
        types of disorders 67
    luteinizing hormone 126
    problems in women 67-79
    retention 80
    stones 77
    symptoms in women 67
    tract infection 77
Urine
    analysis 62, 70
    sediments 28
Urodynamic 70
    evaluation of 76
Uroflowmetry 71
    abnormal flow 71*f*
    normal flow 71*f*
Urogenital atrophy 21, 77
Urogenital distress inventory 69
Urogynecology 197
Uterine
    adenomyosis 59
    artery embolization 47, 48, 87-89
    bleeding: abnormal 35-48
        approach to 36
        etiology 35
        incidence 35
        investigations 38
        management 38

medical management of 39*fc*
surgical management of 39*fc*
bleeding, case of true 35
body 4
cancer 193
cavity abnormalities 124
fibroids 88
leiomyomas 50
polyps
hysteroscopy of 187*f*
ultrasonography of 187*f*
tenderness 163
tumors 188
Uterovesical nodularity 60
Uterus
bicornuate 52*f*
didelphous 53
evaluation of 128
normal 51*f*
recanalization/abnormalities of 52*f*

V

Vagina 6
fecal contamination of 26
flora normally present in 25
natural defense mechanism of 25
organisms normally present in 25
pH of 24
Vaginal
atrophy 196
hysteroscopy of 187*f*
ultrasonography of 187*f*
bleeding 163
candidiasis 26
cells with *Lactobacillus* 29*f*
colonization 21
cream
butoconazole 31
terconazole 31
devices 73
discharge 24, 27, 33
abnormal 24, 26
causes of 26
common causes of 33
normal 24
dryness 196
ecosystems 26
hysterectomy 83

infections, characteristics of 33, 34*t*
pessaries 26
skin 25
suppository terconazole 31
vault cytology 225
Varicocele 137
Vascular
insufficiency 69
invasion 232
Vasomotor symptoms 20
Vasovasostomy 138
Venous thromboembolism 151
Vesicovaginal fistulas 68, 69, 215
Vitamin D 87
Voiding diary 70
Voiding dysfunction 67, 76
causes 76
evaluation 76
treatment 77
Vulva 6, 184
Vulval disease 77
Vulvar cancer 184
Vulvovaginal candidiasis 113
Vulvovaginitis 35

W

Weight loss 72
Wet smear 28
Whiff test 28
White blood cells 34
Willi syndrome 6
Women's contraceptive choices 141
World Health Organization 19, 21, 113, 131, 131*t*, 156
medical eligibility criteria 149
safe abortion guidelines 2012 162*b*

Y

Yasmin 142
Y-chromosome microdeletion 133
Yeast 26
Yuzpe regimen 145

Z

Zerogen tablets 144
Zoladex implant 85
Zoledronic acid 246